ANATOMY OF THE VOICE

OTHER BOOKS BY THEODORE DIMON

Anatomy in Action

Neurodynamics

Your Body, Your Voice

A New Model of Man's Conscious Development

The Body in Motion

Anatomy of the Moving Body, Second Edition

The Elements of Skill

The Undivided Self

ANATOMY OF THE VOICE

An Illustrated Guide
for Singers, Vocal Coaches,
and Speech Therapists

THEODORE DIMON

Illustrated by

G. DAVID BROWN

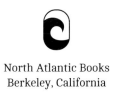

North Atlantic Books
Berkeley, California

Published by
North Atlantic Books
Huichin, unceded Ohlone land
Berkeley, California

Cover art and all illustrations by G. David Brown
Cover design by Howie Severson
Interior book design by G. David Brown

Printed in the United States of America

Anatomy of the Voice: An Illustrated Guide for Singers, Vocal Coaches, and Speech Therapists is sponsored and published by North Atlantic Books, an educational nonprofit based in the unceded Ohlone land Huichin (Berkeley, CA) that collaborates with partners to develop cross-cultural perspectives; nurture holistic views of art, science, the humanities, and healing; and seed personal and global transformation by publishing work on the relationship of body, spirit, and nature.

MEDICAL DISCLAIMER: The following information is intended for general information purposes only. Individuals should always see their health care provider before administering any suggestions made in this book. Any application of the material set forth in the following pages is at the reader's discretion and is their sole responsibility.

North Atlantic Books's publications are distributed to the US trade and internationally by Penguin Random House Publisher Services. For further information, visit our website at www.northatlanticbooks.com.

Library of Congress Cataloging-in-Publication Data

Names: Dimon, Theodore, Jr., author. | Brown, G. David, illustrator.
Title: Anatomy of the voice : an illustrated guide for singers, vocal
  coaches, and speech therapists / Theodore Dimon; illustrated by G. David
  Brown.
Description: Berkeley, California : North Atlantic Books, [2018] | Includes
  index.
Identifiers: LCCN 2017046674 | ISBN 9781623171971 (trade paper)
Subjects: | MESH: Larynx—anatomy & histology | Larynx—physiology | Work of
  Breathing | Voice
Classification: LCC QP306 | NLM WV 501 | DDC 612.2/33—dc23
LC record available at https://lccn.loc.gov/2017046674

6 7 8 9 10 Versa 26 25 24

North Atlantic Books is committed to the protection of our environment. We print on recycled paper whenever possible and partner with printers who strive to use environmentally responsible practices.

TABLE OF CONTENTS

LIST OF ILLUSTRATIONS ix

INTRODUCTION xiii

1. THE ANATOMY OF BREATHING.. 1

The Spine and Rib Cage.. 3

Joints of the Ribs 4

Action of the Ribs... 6

Intercostal Muscles 7

The Diaphragm 10

Action of the Diaphragm... 12

Diaphragm and Abdominal Cavity... 13

The Abdominal Muscles 14

Auxiliary Muscles of Breathing 16

Extensor and Flexor Support of the Trunk.. 17

The Lungs and Trachea 22

Lung Capacity 24

2. THE LARYNX 25

Basic Structure of the Larynx 26

The Framework of the Larynx 27

The Epiglottis... 28

Cricoarytenoid Joint 28

Cricothyroid Joint 29

Conus Elasticus 30

The Interior of the Larynx... 30

Muscles of the Epiglottis 32

The Structure of the Vocal Folds 34

Intrinsic Muscles of the Larynx 34

Actions of the Intrinsic Muscles of the Larynx 37

Cricothyroid and Thyroarytenoid Antagonism.. 42

Action of the Larynx Muscles in Chest Register 43

Action of the Larynx Muscles in Falsetto Register.................................... 44

Action of the Larynx Muscles in Head Register....................................... 45

3. THE EXTRINSIC MUSCLES OF THE LARYNX 47

The Suspensory Muscles of the Larynx 48

Action of the Suspensory Muscles during Singing 51

Supported Falsetto 53

Head Voice 53

The Hyoid Apparatus 54

Sidebar: The Hyoid Bone 55

Muscles of the Hyoid Bone and Jaw 56

4. THE MOUTH AND PHARYNX 59

Muscles of the Mouth and Throat 61

The Function of the Palate 63

The Muscles of the Palate 64

Sidebar: The Action of Swallowing (Deglutition) 66

The Arched Palate 66

The Tongue and Its Function 68

Position of the Tongue in Singing 69

The Low Larynx and Widened Pharynx 71

5. THE FACE AND JAW 73

The Mask 74

The Nostrils and Nasal Cavity 75

Muscles of the Nostrils 76

The Eyes and Forehead 78

The Cheeks 80

The Jaw and Temporomandibular Joint 82

Position of the Jaw in Singing 83

Muscles of the Jaw 84

6. THE EVOLUTION AND FUNCTION OF THE LARYNX 87

The Origin of the Larynx 87

Evolution of the Cartilages and Muscles of the Larynx 88

Extrinsic Muscles of the Larynx and Deglutition 88

The Palate, Epiglottis, and Nasal Passages 90

Design of the Vocal Folds 92

The Pharynx, Upright Posture, and Human Speech 94

EPILOGUE 97

INDEX 99

ABOUT THE AUTHOR 103

LIST OF ILLUSTRATIONS

1. THE ANATOMY OF BREATHING

1-1. Movement of the rib cage

1-2. Movement of the diaphragm

1-3. Rib cage and spine

1-4. Diaphragm as partition between thoracic and abdominal contents

1-5. Costovertebral or rib joint of T5

1-6. Types of ribs

1-7. Ribs move like the handles of a pail

1-8. Action of rib at joint: a. Sagittal section of rib joint; b. Range of motion of rib

1-9. External and internal intercostal muscles

1-10. Levatores costarum, levator costae, and quadratus lumborum

1-11. Transversus thoracis muscle

1-12. The diaphragm

1-13. Diaphragm showing placement of heart on top, as well as viscera below, which are pushed down in inhalation

1-14. Front and side views of diaphragm and its movements during breathing

1-15. Diaphragm descending

1-16. Diaphragm descending and ribs ascending

1-17. Action of diaphragm in relation to rib movement (assisting in elevating ribs)

1-18. Intercostals and obliques of trunk

1-19. a. External abdominal oblique muscle; b. Internal abdominal oblique muscle; c. Transversalis

1-20. Rectus abdominis muscle

1-21. Sternocleidomastoid muscle

1-22. Scalene muscles

1-23. a. Deep postural muscles; b. Sacrospinalis group

1-24. Flexor support of sternocleidomastoid and rectus abdominis muscles

1-25. Third layer: serratus muscles

1-26. Fourth layer: scapula muscles

1-27. Fifth layer: trapezius and latissimus dorsi

1-28. The lungs and trachea

1-29. a. Total lung capacity; b. Lung capacity in relaxed state

2. THE LARYNX

2-1. a. Vocal folds open; b. Vocal folds closed; c. Vocal folds approximated for phonation

2-2. Cartilages and vocal folds

2-3. The framework of the larynx

2-4. Thyroid, cricoid, and arytenoid cartilages

2-5. Cricoarytenoid joint: a. Articular facets on cricoid; b. Movement of arytenoid cartilages on the cricoid cartilage

2-6. Cricothyroid joint

2-7. Conus elasticus

2-8. The interior of the larynx

2-9. The aryepiglottic muscle of the epiglottis

2-10. The thyroepiglottic muscle of the epiglottis

2-11. Cricothyroid muscle

2-12. Vocalis and thyroarytenoid muscles

2-13. The glottis.

2-14. The posterior cricoarytenoid muscle

2-15. The lateral cricoarytenoid muscle

2-16. The transverse and oblique arytenoid muscles

2-17. Action of the posterior cricoarytenoid muscles, the openers

2-18. Action of the lateral cricoarytenoid muscles, which close the glottis

2-19. Action of transverse and oblique arytenoid muscles, which close the glottis
2-20. The cricothyroid, a stretching muscle
2-21. Stretching of the vocal folds
2-22. Tensors of the larynx
2-23. Wave action of the vocal folds
2-24. Vocal folds in chest voice
2-25. Vocal folds in falsetto

3. THE EXTRINSIC MUSCLES OF THE LARYNX

3-1. Suspensory muscles of the larynx
3-2. Base of skull with styloid and mastoid process
3-3. Complete suspensory muscles of the larynx
3-4. a. Elevation of larynx in singing; b. Strained appearance of singer; c. Lines of force of the elevators
3-5. Action of the suspensory muscles during singing
3-6. Action of suspensory muscles in supported falsetto
3-7. Action of suspensory muscles in head voice
3-8. Hyoid apparatus
3-9. Styloid process and hyoid bone
3-10. Complete hyoid muscles
3-11. False elevators of tongue
3-12. The strap muscles

4. THE MOUTH AND PHARYNX

4-1. The vocal tract
4-2. The articulators
4-3. Muscles of the mouth and throat
4-4. Constrictors of the throat
4-5. Valve action of the palate: a. Velopharyngeal closure of soft palate against back of pharynx; b. Oral seal formed by back of tongue contacting soft palate; c. Both actions combining to seal nasal and oral passages
4-6. Elevators of the palate
4-7. Depressors of palate
4-8. The soft palate: a. Arched; b. Depressed
4-9. The tongue and its muscles
4-10. a. Position of the tongue during singing: open throat; b. Raised position of tongue: closed throat
4-11. Position of the tongue in vowel formation
4-12. a. Raised larynx and constricted throat; b. Lowered larynx and open throat

5. THE FACE AND JAW

5-1. Muscles of the face
5-2. The mask
5-3. Nasal cavity
5-4. Muscles of the nose
5-5. Muscles of the eyes and forehead
5-6. Muscles of the cheek and mouth
5-7. The jaw and temporomandibular joint
5-8. a. Partial opening of the jaw for speaking: hinge action; b. Wider opening of the jaw for singing: hinge and gliding action
5-9. Muscles of the jaw
5-10. Depressors of the jaw
5-11. The diaphragm of the jaw

6. THE EVOLUTION AND FUNCTION OF THE LARYNX

6-1.   The larynx functions as a sphincter to close off the airway

6-2.   Sphincter muscles and dilator

6-3.   The muscles that dilate and close the airway

6-4.   Palate and separation of nasal and oral passageway: a. Reptile; b. Mammal

6-5.   Epiglottis and palate in herbivore showing how the epiglottis links with the palate to close off mouth to breathing

6-6.   a. & b. Coronal view of larynx showing inlet and outlet valves (ventricular bands and vocal folds); c. The vocal folds do not oppose the outflow of air and vibrate to produce sound

6-7.   Pharynx as resonator in: a. Apes; b. Man

INTRODUCTION

This book has been written as a reference for singers, vocal coaches, speech therapists, and students of voice who require detailed information on the anatomy of the voice and how it works. Although many books on singing and speech are currently available, very few of them actually present the basic anatomy of the voice in clear and simple terms, which is the aim of this work. Readers familiar with my first book on the voice, *Your Body, Your Voice,* will know that I have already presented a new approach to the subject of voice production. This new book complements the first volume, in which the basics of anatomy of the voice were not included.

In compiling basic anatomical information on the voice, the first question that arises is what to include. In this book I have identified five basic systems that are responsible for vocal production:

The first, and in many ways the most basic part of the voice, is the respiratory system. Although sound is produced in the larynx, this would not be possible without the flow of air from the lungs. This airflow provides a necessary power source to set the vocal cords into motion to produce sound. In Chapter One we'll look at the anatomy of breathing.

Chapter Two examines the second system, the larynx, which is the most immediate physical structure pertaining to the voice. Its role in vocal production and its highly specialized functions are so important that it merits a key place in a basic anatomical reference on the voice. The larynx forms the housing for the vocal folds that vibrate to make sound, bringing them together when we want to speak or sing, and pulling them apart when we breathe normally. Though the intricate design of the larynx does not lend itself to easy comprehension of its function, when we break down its component parts and look at them in turn, it begins to make sense.

The larynx itself is suspended within a network of muscles—sometimes called the extrinsic muscles of the larynx—that move the structure when we swallow and help it to function. These constitute the third system we will examine. Although the role of these muscles in swallowing is well understood, their role in vocalization has been largely misunderstood and underestimated. We'll look at the function of these muscles in Chapter Three.

The fourth basic system is the vocal tract, which is made up mainly of the pharynx but also includes the oral cavity and the position of the larynx. It is here that we break up the sounds coming from the larynx into speech. It is also here that the sound from the vibrating vocal folds is augmented. Because the vocal tract is not fixed in shape but can be altered by how we use the different structures such as the mouth, tongue, and palate, it forms a crucial part of vocal training. We'll look at these elements in detail in Chapter Four.

Because the face also occupies a practical role in vocal training, I have included a fifth chapter describing the muscles of the face as they relate to vocal placement. Here I have also included the jaw, since it naturally belongs in this section.

In the final chapter we will look at the function and evolution of the larynx in particular, and the voice in general. Because the larynx is so complex, it is nearly impossible to appreciate why it is the way it is without having some sense of how it evolved, which in turn helps to make some of its features more understandable.

CHAPTER 1

THE ANATOMY OF BREATHING

*B*reathing is one of the most vital of our life processes. All day long, throughout our lives, we take in air in order to provide cells throughout the body with oxygen and then expel carbon dioxide from the lungs in order to rid the body of wastes produced by cellular activity. Secondarily, breathing is the power source that sets the vocal folds into motion to produce sound. To do this, we do not exhale normally but alter our breathing so that we can produce the sustained sounds of speech and song.

Although breathing refers to the flow of air into and out of our bodies, we actually breathe by altering the size of our chest cavity, not by doing something to the air. By making the space within the chest cavity get larger and smaller, air flows into and out of the chest through either the nose or mouth. That simple exchange of air is what we call breathing.

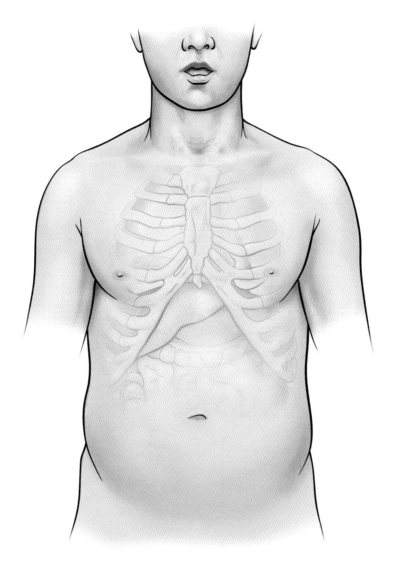

There are two ways that we increase and decrease the size of the chest cavity. First, the ribs, which form the chest cavity, are capable of rising like pail handles by moving at the joints where they attach to the spine; this action increases the space within the chest (Fig. 1-1). The uppermost ribs connect in front to the sternum; those below form an arch beneath it; the last two, the floating ribs, do not attach in front. Because of this, not all the ribs move in the same way, or to the same degree. But most of the ribs rise and widen to some extent, making the space inside the chest larger; when they return to their lower position, the space gets smaller.

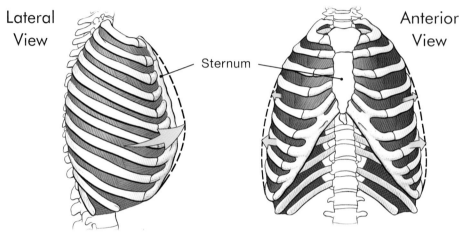

Figure 1-1. Movement of the rib cage.

Second, the bottom of the thoracic cavity is separated from the abdominal contents below by the dome-like muscle of the diaphragm, which, by contracting, can flatten out and thus increase the size of the lower part of the chest cavity (Fig. 1-2). When the ribs rise and open, the diaphragm contracts and descends; the chest cavity increases and air rushes in to fill the lungs. When the ribs return to normal position, the diaphragm relaxes and ascends, air is forced out, and we exhale.

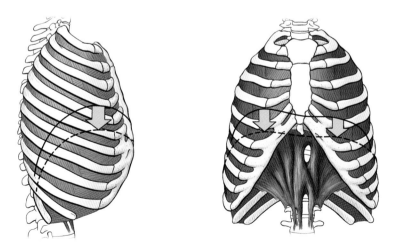

Figure 1-2. Movement of the diaphragm.

The Spine and Rib Cage

The basic framework for the respiratory system is the spine and rib cage. The spine is made up of twenty-four vertebrae—five in the lumbar region, twelve in the thoracic, and seven in the cervical. There is a rib on each side of the twelve thoracic vertebrae, forming the rib cage (Fig. 1-3).

There are twelve ribs on each side of the body that correspond to the twelve thoracic vertebrae of the spine. The first seven attach in front to the sternum, or breastbone; these are called true ribs. The remaining five are called false ribs because they do not attach directly to the sternum, but join each other to form an arch called the costal arch, which can be easily felt below the sternum. The final two ribs are called the floating ribs because they do not attach in front. The ribs attaching to the sternum and the costal arch are not bony all the way around. At their extremity the bone becomes cartilage, so that the connection of the ribs with the sternum and the costal arch is cartilaginous and quite flexible. The costal arch is also made up of cartilage.

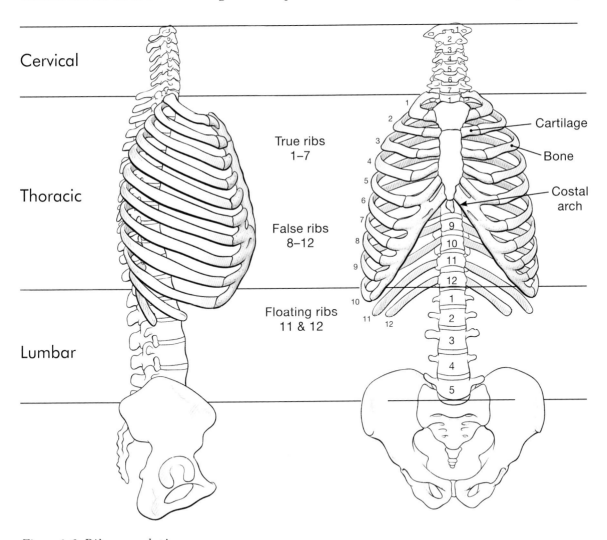

Figure 1-3. Rib cage and spine.

Within the rib cage are the lungs and heart. The heart sits right behind the lower part of the sternum and a little to the left; the lungs are on either side of the heart. The diaphragm forms the lower boundary of the thorax (Fig. 1-4); the heart and lungs lie above the diaphragm, and all the other major internal organs lie below the diaphragm, which forms a boundary between these upper and lower regions of the trunk. "Diaphragm" is actually a descriptive term that the Greeks gave to this muscle: it means "a partition wall."

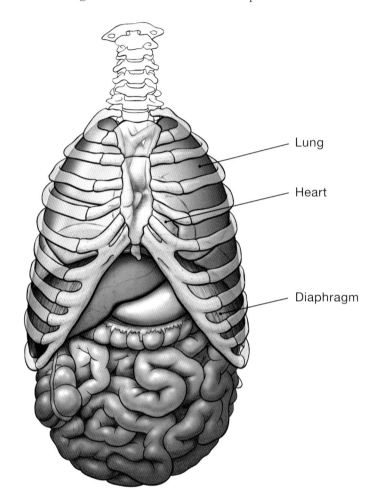

Figure 1–4. Diaphragm as partition between thoracic and abdominal contents.

Joints of the Ribs

Each of the twelve ribs moves in relation to the spine, where they form the costovertebral joints (Fig. 1-5). Each rib articulates with the spine in several places. First, the head of the rib articulates with the lower part of the body of one vertebra and the upper part of the one below it, as well as with the disc in between the two vertebrae. Second, the neck of the rib articulates with the transverse process of the lower of these two vertebrae.

The rib is firmly bound at each of these articulations by several ligaments, permitting a limited rotation at the joint that nevertheless translates into quite a lot of movement over the entire length of the rib. Some of the ribs have simpler articulations, but the main thing to keep in mind is that the ribs actually articulate at the spine to permit the movements essential to breathing.

At the front part of the rib cage the ribs terminate and become cartilaginous. This allows a measure of flexibility in the front of the ribs. The sections where bone becomes cartilage form gliding joints that permit the ribs some movement in relation to the sternum so that both the sternum and ribs have a certain degree of movement in front as the ribs rise and fall.

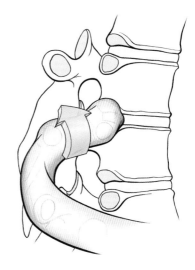

Figure 1-5. Costovertebral or rib joint of T5.

The ribs are not all identical in character (Fig. 1-6). The topmost rib is short, flat, and round. We often think of the upper ribs as being almost as large as the middle ones. However, the topmost rib, which forms the opening into the thorax, or thoracic inlet, is quite small—only a third the width of the shoulder girdle. It is through this opening that the windpipe, esophagus, and other structures pass from the neck down into the chest. The next rib is larger but shaped rather like the first. Going downward, the ribs increase in length until the seventh rib, after which they begin to get smaller again. They also slant down obliquely, corresponding to the muscles of the trunk, which also slant and spiral around the trunk. The final two floating ribs, which are much shorter than the ones above, are very flexible in their movements because they do not attach to anything in front; their function is mainly to provide attachments for the diaphragm.

In back, the ribs do not extend directly to the sides to form the rib cage; they actually angle backward almost to the level of the spinous processes of the vertebrae. This means that there is a gap between the spinous processes and the posterior part of the rib on either side. This gap is filled up with the longitudinal extensor muscles, which give the back a flat appearance.

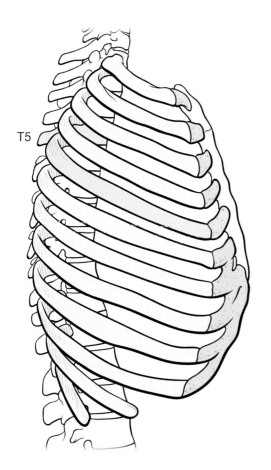

T5

Figure 1-6. Types of ribs.

Action of the Ribs

The movement of the ribs is crucial to breathing. Because the ribs slant down at an oblique angle, they hang below the point where they articulate with the spine. When we inhale, the ribs, by rotating where they articulate with the spine, move like pail handles being raised slightly (Fig. 1-7). This rotation raises the sides of the ribs, which increases the lateral dimension of the thorax. It also brings the front of the rib forward as it moves upward, which increases the anteroposterior dimensions of the thorax as well (Fig. 1-8). These movements increase the space within the thorax, causing air to flow into the lungs. Of course, not all the ribs move in the same way: the first ribs move very little, and there is in general more movement as you go lower down. The final two floating ribs, which are not attached either directly or indirectly to the sternum, have even greater mobility.

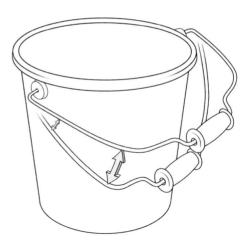

Figure 1-7. Ribs move like the handles of a pail.

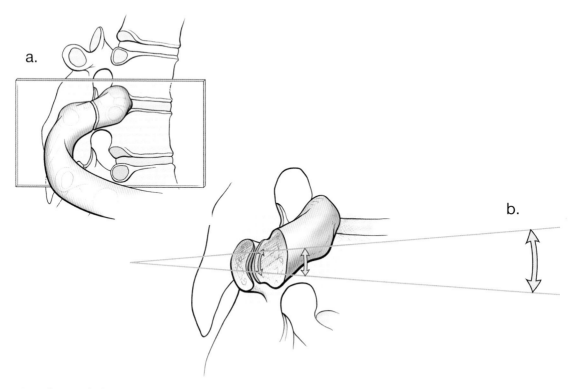

Figure 1-8. Action of rib at joint: a. Sagittal section of rib joint; b. Range of motion of rib.

Intercostal Muscles

There are two layers of rib, or intercostal muscles that are directly responsible for respiratory movements of the ribs in breathing (Fig. 1-9). There are eleven external intercostal muscles, one between each of the twelve ribs. They originate at the lower border of each rib and attach to the upper border of the rib below, running obliquely down and forward. Underneath this layer are the eleven internal intercostal muscles that originate at the inner surface of each rib and slant down and back, in the opposite direction to the external intercostals, to attach to the rib below.

The external intercostals function mainly to elevate the ribs, increasing the width of the thoracic cavity and causing inspiration. You can see from the angle of the muscle what the effect of contraction will be. When the upper ribs are held or fixed in place by the scalene muscles above (see Fig. 1-22), the contracting fibers pull from above to raise the ribs below, increasing the overall capacity of the chest.

Conversely, the internal intercostals act in the opposite direction, depressing the ribs when they contract, actively facilitating breathing out.

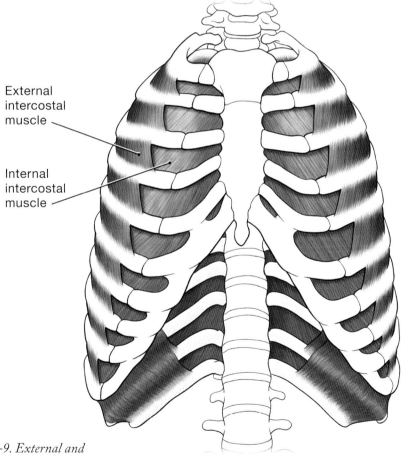

External
intercostal
muscle

Internal
intercostal
muscle

Figure 1-9. External and internal intercostal muscles.

The levatores costarum and levator costae muscles originate at the transverse processes of the vertebrae and, running obliquely downward, attach to the ribs below (Fig. 1-10). These muscles, as their name suggests, assist the external intercostals in raising the ribs. When the quadratus lumborum muscle and levatores costarum are functioning properly, the lower back becomes elastic and filled out, and the floating ribs move freely. This coordinated lengthening and widening in the back tends to lend greater mobility to the ribs, which can then expand and move more freely.

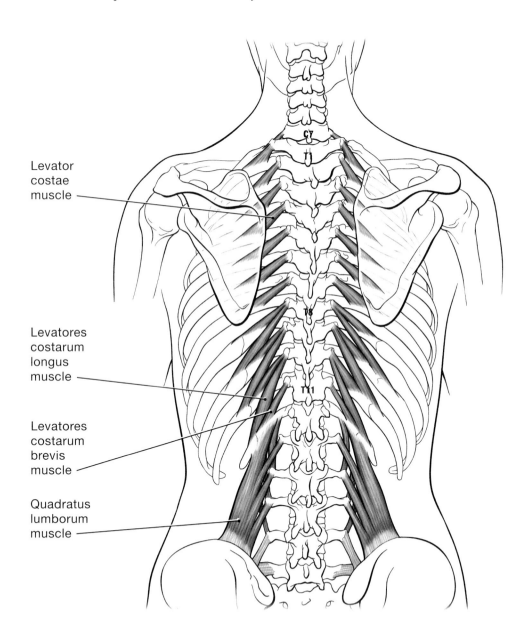

Levator
costae
muscle

Levatores
costarum
longus
muscle

Levatores
costarum
brevis
muscle

Quadratus
lumborum
muscle

Figure 1-10. Levatores costarum, levator costae, and quadratus lumborum.

The transversus thoracis muscle lies on the inner surface of the lower part of the sternum (Fig. 1-11). Its fibers extend up and out, like the splayed fingers of a hand, and insert into the costal cartilages of the second, third, fourth, fifth, and sixth ribs. This muscle, which when contracted aids in forceful expiration, is the muscle that you can sometimes feel gripping in the inner chest; it contributes to the rigidity of the chest in many people who raise and fix the chest when speaking and breathing.

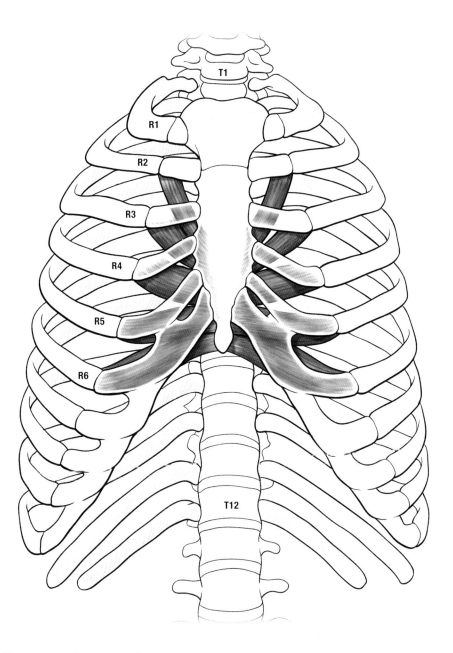

Figure 1-11. Transversus thoracis muscle.

The Diaphragm

The diaphragm is the main muscle of breathing (Fig. 1-12). It is a large, dome-shaped muscle that divides the thoracic and abdominal cavities (as we saw earlier, the word "diaphragm" means "partition wall"). Its muscular fibers arise from the anterior spine and the entire circumference of the lower thorax and converge upward into a central tendinous peak that forms two domes on either side of this central tendon. Its largest and lowest origin is a tendon called the crus, which originates from both sides of the lumbar spine, so that the muscle appears to fan upward from the lower spine.

The other portions of the diaphragm arise from a tendon at the lower part of the sternum, from the costal arch formed by the lowest six or seven ribs, and from a ligament that spans the lower back from the first or second lumbar vertebra to the lowest floating rib. From these points the muscular fibers of the diaphragm ascend in an arch to form a central tendinous aponeurosis at its top. The heart sits directly on top of the diaphragm, nestled between the lungs on either side. The fibers of the pericardium, the membrane that encloses the heart, intermingle with those of this central tendon so that the two are actually attached. The central tendon also extends to the sides, forming the top of each dome, so that the central tendinous sheet on the top of the diaphragm has three sections, or leaflets.

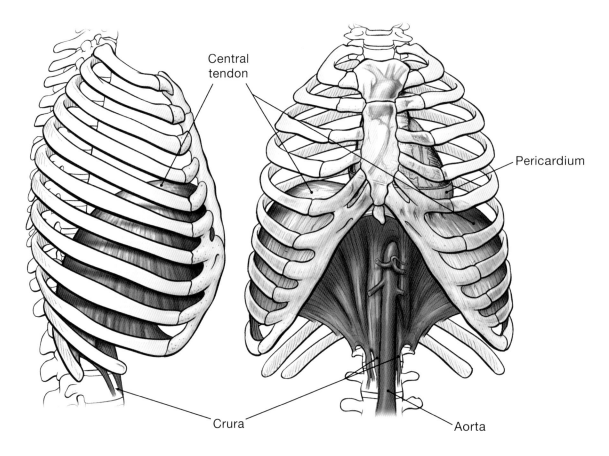

Figure 1-12. The diaphragm.

Because the diaphragm forms the upper boundary of the abdominal region, it quite literally sits above the viscera—the liver on the right side and the stomach and spleen on the left (Fig. 1-13). The shape of the diaphragm is actually a double dome, the right dome being higher than the left to accommodate the liver, so that it appears as a somewhat lopsided mushroom. It is penetrated by the aorta, the esophagus, and the vena cava (the large blood vessel that returns blood to the heart), which pass from the chest into the abdominal region. The normal resting height of the domes of the diaphragm at their highest point is roughly on a level with the fifth rib. During deep inhalation, the domes descend one to two inches, roughly to the level of the bottom of the sternum (see Fig. 1-2).

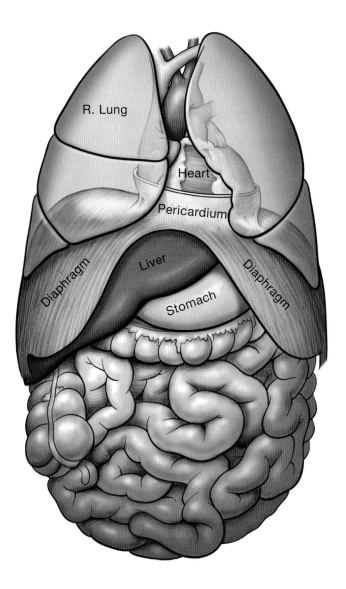

Figure 1–13. Diaphragm showing placement of heart on top, as well as viscera below, which are pushed down in inhalation.

Action of the Diaphragm

The diaphragm is an extremely active and hardworking muscle that contracts rhythmically every few seconds during normal breathing to ensure a constant supply of air to the lungs. As we have seen, the entire top section of the diaphragm is composed of tendinous tissue and is therefore passive. The contractile portion of the diaphragm is formed by the muscular fibers that pass downward from this central tendinous sheet around its entire circumference to their origins around the circumference of the thorax. When the diaphragm contracts, these muscular fibers tend to flatten out the central tendon and draw it downward; this increases the space in the lower thorax and causes air to flow into the lungs (Figs. 1-14 and 1-15). At the same time, the ribs ascend, which also contributes to the expansion of the space within the chest cavity and the flow of air into the lungs (Fig. 1-16). Note that the active movement of the diaphragm is downward, not upward as many people mistakenly think (perhaps because the ribs go up in inhalation). The diaphragm does not contribute to the exhalation of air or directly "support" the breath; it returns to its higher position as a result of the elastic recoil of its muscular fibers.

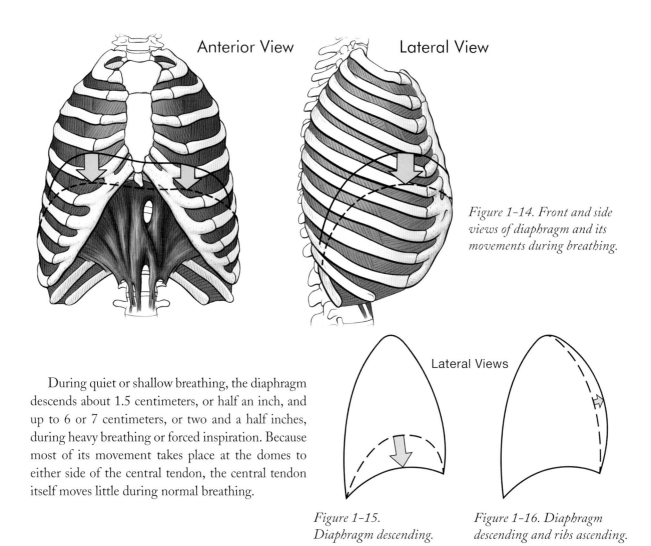

Anterior View   Lateral View

Figure 1-14. Front and side views of diaphragm and its movements during breathing.

During quiet or shallow breathing, the diaphragm descends about 1.5 centimeters, or half an inch, and up to 6 or 7 centimeters, or two and a half inches, during heavy breathing or forced inspiration. Because most of its movement takes place at the domes to either side of the central tendon, the central tendon itself moves little during normal breathing.

Lateral Views

Figure 1-15. Diaphragm descending.

Figure 1-16. Diaphragm descending and ribs ascending.

Diaphragm and Abdominal Cavity

Because the diaphragm sits on top of the abdominal cavity, its action is affected by the contents of the abdomen and the abdominal muscles. The abdomen acts somewhat like a flexible, fluid-filled container. When the diaphragm contracts, its descent forces the contents of the abdomen outward, particularly if the abdomen is relaxed. If the abdominal muscles contract, however, the viscera cannot move outward and the diaphragm is restricted in its downward movement. The central tendon then acts as a fixed point from which the lower ribs are pulled on by the contracting muscular fibers of the diaphragm, thus elevating them and expanding the lower thoracic cavity (Fig. 1-17). The abdominal muscles can thus assist the action of the diaphragm; however, singers who are overly preoccupied with getting breath or who use excessive effort to try to support the breath can end up overworking the diaphragm, which becomes chronically contracted. This has the effect over time of distending the ribs and distorting the lower rib cage.

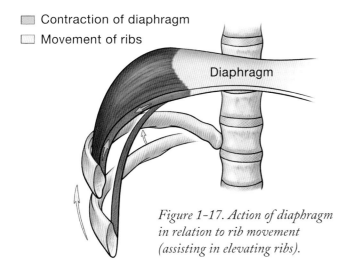

☐ Contraction of diaphragm
☐ Movement of ribs

Diaphragm

Figure 1-17. Action of diaphragm in relation to rib movement (assisting in elevating ribs).

In normal breathing, inhalation is active and exhalation is passive. When we breathe in, the ribs are raised and the diaphragm actively lowers as muscle contraction occurs. When we breathe out, the thoracic walls and diaphragm, as well as the expanded lung tissue, elastically recoil and passively force air out of the lungs. In contrast, when we forcefully expel air from the lungs, contraction of the internal intercostals and the abdominal muscles actively compress the ribs, forcing the air out.

During vocalization, muscles of both inhalation and exhalation are active. When we take air into the lungs and are about to breathe out, the tendency for air to rush out of the lungs is so great that, in order to counterbalance this force and to produce a controlled flow of air suitable for phonation, inspiratory forces must actively counterbalance passive recoil forces. To accomplish this, the internal intercostal muscles and diaphragm maintain tone and recoil slowly to their resting state in order to control the outflow of air. The action of the diaphragm also opposes the descent of the ribs, particularly if the exhalation muscles are actively working to press air out. The diaphragm thus counteracts the out-breathing tendency by maintaining the expansion of the ribs to help "support" the breath.

The muscles of expiration also come into play in singing if the lungs and thorax have recoiled to their resting size and the singer still needs to produce sound; in this case, abdominal and thoracic expiratory muscles are actively employed in helping to contract the ribs and to press the viscera up against the diaphragm, thus expelling more air.

The Abdominal Muscles

The muscles in the abdominal region are continuous with those of the ribs, running in corresponding oblique directions (Fig. 1-18). There are three layers of abdominal muscles, corresponding to the external and internal intercostal muscles and the transversus thoracis, the muscle underlying the sternum. The external abdominal oblique muscle originates at the eight lowest ribs; its fibers run downward to attach to the rim of the pelvis, or iliac crest, and obliquely downward and forward to end in aponeurotic tissue that terminates at the linea alba (Fig. 1-19a). This muscle is continuous with the external intercostal muscle of the thorax.

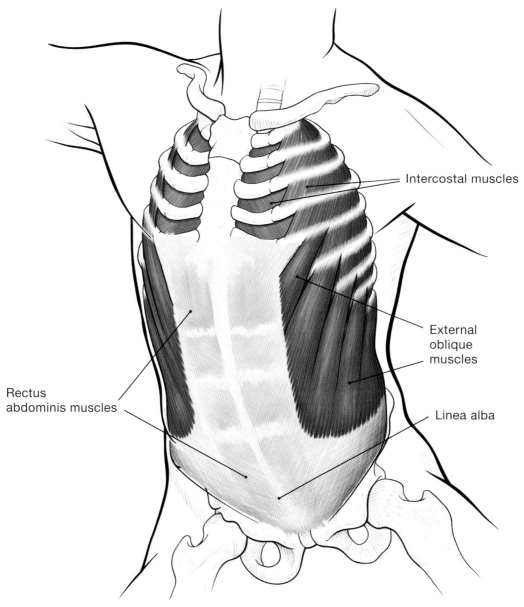

Intercostal muscles

External oblique muscles

Rectus abdominis muscles

Linea alba

Figure 1-18. Intercostals and obliques of trunk.

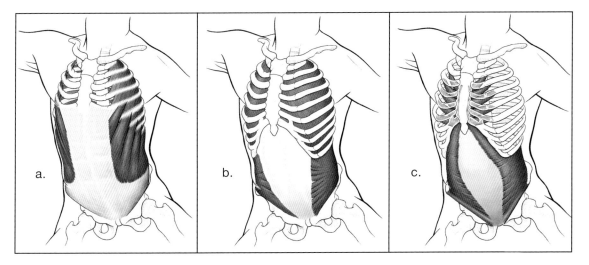

Figure 1-19. a. External abdominal oblique muscle; b. Internal abdominal oblique muscle; c. Transversalis muscle.

The internal abdominal oblique muscle originates at the inguinal ligament, the iliac crest, and the lumbar fascia (Fig. 1-19b). Its fibers fan out to attach to the pubic bone, the linea alba, and the lower three ribs. It is continuous with the internal intercostal muscle of the thorax.

The third and deepest muscle, corresponding to the transversus thoracis muscle of the chest, is the transversus abdominis, or transversalis (Fig. 1-19c). It originates at the crest of the ilium, the lumbar fascia, and the ribs and runs, as its name suggests, horizontally around the midriff. It terminates in aponeurotic tissue, joining the linea alba and the pubic symphysis.

Rectus abdominis is the longitudinal muscle vertically spanning the front of the abdomen (Fig. 1-20). It originates at the pubic symphysis and runs vertically up each side of the linea alba at a slightly outward angle to insert into the fifth, sixth, and seventh ribs; it is enclosed within a sheath of tendon formed by the oblique and transversalis muscles. By acting on the rib cage, this muscle powerfully contracts or flexes the front of the body (as in performing a sit-up); it also powerfully contracts the lower part of the rib cage.

All the abdominal muscles are actively engaged during forceful expiration of air. During vocalization, the diaphragm does not relax all at once but maintains tension so that air is released slowly; as we just saw, the abdominal muscles maintain tension of the abdominal cavity in conjunction with the action of the diaphragm.

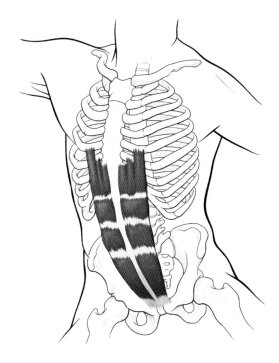

Figure 1-20. Rectus abdominis muscle.

Auxiliary Muscles of Breathing

There are several auxiliary muscles of breathing. The first is the sternocleidomastoid muscle (Fig. 1-21), which originates by two heads at the sternum and clavicle and attaches to the mastoid process of the skull. This muscle is a flexor of the head and neck, and assists in rotation of the head. Like the scalene muscles, it is considered an accessory muscle in breathing and noticeably contracts during forced inspiration.

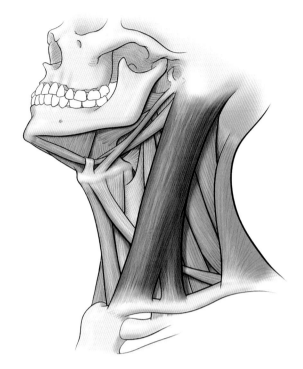

Figure 1-21. Sternocleidomastoid muscle.

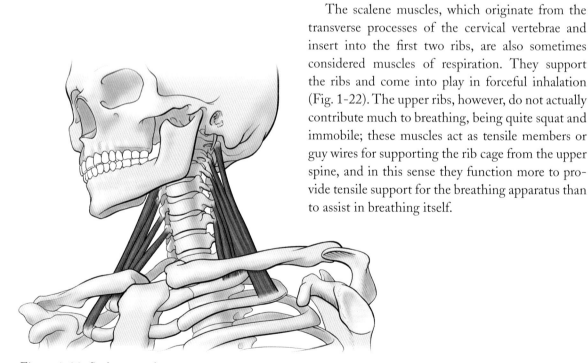

Figure 1-22. Scalene muscles.

The scalene muscles, which originate from the transverse processes of the cervical vertebrae and insert into the first two ribs, are also sometimes considered muscles of respiration. They support the ribs and come into play in forceful inhalation (Fig. 1-22). The upper ribs, however, do not actually contribute much to breathing, being quite squat and immobile; these muscles act as tensile members or guy wires for supporting the rib cage from the upper spine, and in this sense they function more to provide tensile support for the breathing apparatus than to assist in breathing itself.

Extensor and Flexor Support of the Trunk

Although the intercostal muscles are the prime movers of the ribs during breathing, the correct working of our overall upright support system is the essential foundation of coordinated breathing. This system can be divided into three functional groups of which the most important is composed of the two deepest layers of postural muscles that support the trunk as a whole. The first and deepest layer is composed of the small postural muscles that act upon the vertebrae along the entire length of the spine; their function is to maintain the elongation and support of the spine. The second layer comprises the sacrospinalis or erector spinae muscles, which form large meaty bundles attaching to the ribs and running vertically up the length of the spine. Their function is to maintain the erect posture of the trunk by keeping it from buckling forward. The proper working of these muscles ensures that the ribs are able to move freely; if they are overly tense, their constriction will fix the ribs and interfere with breathing (Fig. 1-23).

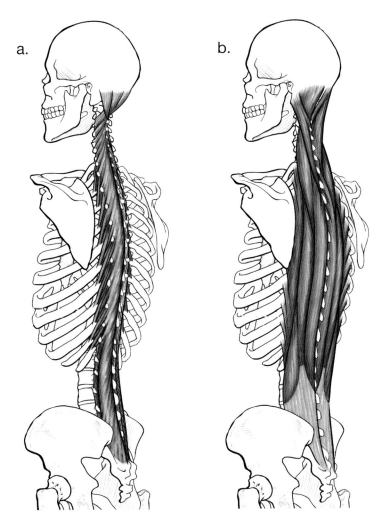

Figure 1-23. a. Deep postural muscles; b. Sacrospinalis group.

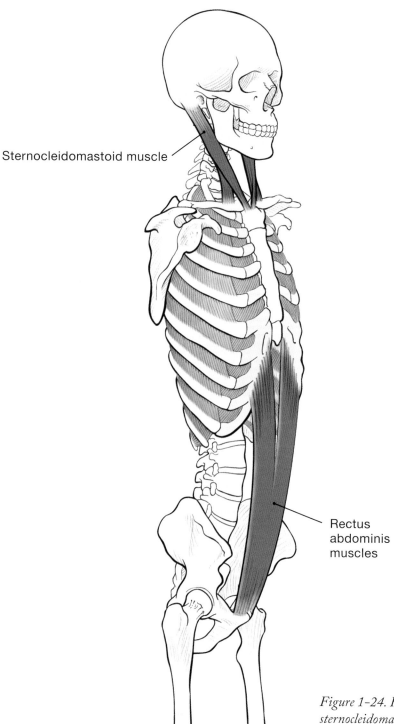

Sternocleidomastoid muscle

Rectus
abdominis
muscles

The second key group of muscles in our upright support system is composed of the sternocleidomastoid muscle and other key anterior flexors such as the rectus abdominis muscle, which provide tensile support for the thorax as a whole. The sternocleidomastoid muscle is a crucial suspensory muscle for the rib cage and the front of the body (Fig. 1-24). In the framework of this support, the intercostals may be considered the intrinsic muscles of breathing: they make the immediate action happen, but function properly only in the context of the larger support network of extensors and flexors that ensure the proper support and mobility of the trunk and rib cage.

Figure 1-24. Flexor support of sternocleidomastoid muscle and rectus abdominis muscles.

The third group comprises the oblique muscles of the back and shoulder girdle, which enable the ribs to move because of their widening action. This group is composed of the third layer of back muscles (Fig. 1-25). Serratus posterior superior originates at the spinous processes of the last cervical and first two thoracic vertebrae and, inclining downward and outward, inserts like four fingers into the second, third, fourth, and fifth ribs. Serratus posterior inferior originates at the spinous processes of the upper lumbar and lower thoracic vertebrae, passes obliquely up and outward, and, breaking like serratus superior into four branches, inserts into the four lower ribs. These muscles act upon the ribs, serratus superior raising the ribs, and serratus inferior drawing the lower ribs down and widening the back. Along with quadratus lumborum (which attaches from the pelvis to the lowest rib and which we'll discuss when we get to the thorax) and levatores costarum (which we've seen is one of the deeper muscles attaching to the transverse processes of the vertebrae), serratus posterior inferior and superior play an important role in freeing the ribs and widening the back. When they are releasing, these muscles contribute to the freedom and fullness of the lower back, as well as the proper working of the diaphragm, which is directly related to the lower ribs.

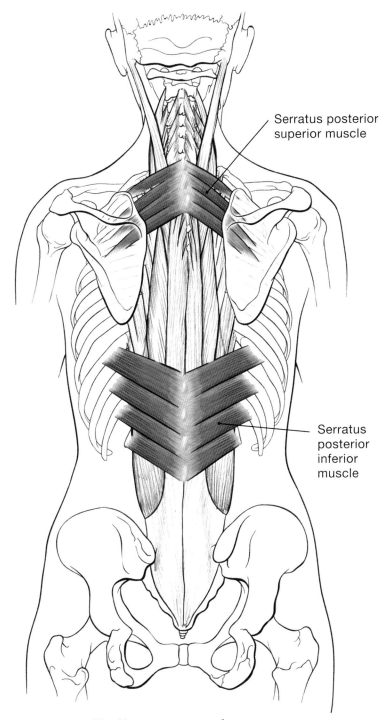

Serratus posterior superior muscle

Serratus posterior inferior muscle

Figure 1-25. Third layer: serratus muscles.

Levator scapulae, rhomboid minor, and rhomboid major act upon the scapulae (Fig. 1-26). Originating at the transverse processes of the atlas and upper cervical vertebrae, levator scapulae attaches to the side of the scapula. This muscle, as its name suggests, elevates the scapula. Rhomboid minor originates at the seventh cervical and first thoracic vertebrae and passes downward and outward to insert into the spine of the scapula. Rhomboid major originates at the spinous processes of the four or five upper thoracic vertebrae and attaches to the lower spine of the scapula. Both of these muscles, which are so named because of their rhomboidal shape, help to stabilize the scapula when the arms are being moved. These layers of back muscles are also crucial for breathing; because they run obliquely and horizontally, their free action ensures the mobility and widening of the ribs.

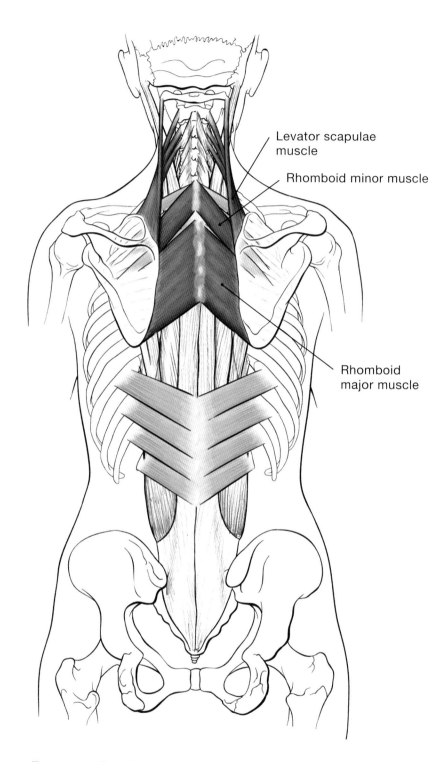

Levator scapulae muscle

Rhomboid minor muscle

Rhomboid major muscle

Figure 1-26. Fourth layer: scapula muscles.

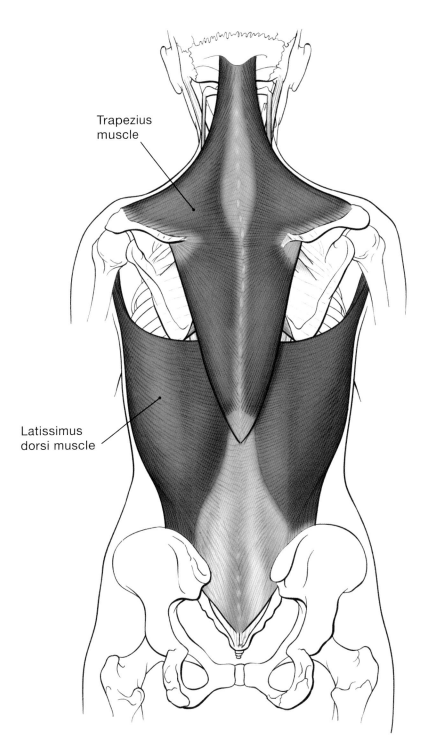

Trapezius muscle

Latissimus dorsi muscle

The most superficial muscle layer of the back consists of two powerful sheets of muscle covering most of the back: these are trapezius and latissimus dorsi (Fig. 1-27). Trapezius is a diamond-shaped muscle covering the neck and upper shoulders. It originates broadly at the occiput and the spinous processes of the cervical and thoracic vertebrae and inserts into the upper scapula and the clavicle. Trapezius acts upon the shoulder blades, retracting them or pulling them together, bracing the shoulder in strong skeletal movements, and elevating the shoulder as in lifting weights. Latissimus dorsi is a broad, flat sheet of muscle covering the lower half of the back and inserting into the humerus, the upper arm bone. It originates at the spinous processes of the sacral, lumbar, and lower thoracic vertebrae, and from this very broad origin converges into the upper arm bone. Latissimus depresses the upper arm, but because it contributes to the widening support of the back, it provides crucial support and elasticity to the action of the ribs and unimpeded breathing.

Figure 1-27. Fifth layer: trapezius and latissimus dorsi.

The Lungs and Trachea

The trachea, or windpipe, extends from the throat downward, and divides into the two bronchial tubes that enter the lungs (Fig. 1-28). It is four or five inches long, and sits in front of the esophagus. It is composed of an elastic fibrous membrane that is reinforced around two-thirds of its circumference by cartilaginous rings (the first of these is sometimes continuous with the cricoid cartilage of the larynx). The trachea is lined with muscular fibers, as well as a mucous membrane that is continuous with the membrane lining the larynx above. At the lower end of the trachea, the two bronchi divide into progressively smaller airways that subdivide to form bronchioles that lead into tiny balloon-like air sacs called alveoli, which is where the oxygen exchange takes place between the lungs and the blood.

The lungs themselves are conical in shape with concave bases that conform to the domes of the diaphragm. The right lung has three lobes and the left, which is smaller to accommodate the heart, only two. Each lung is of a lightweight, spongy texture and weighs a little over a pound, and each is encased within a thin pleura, or membrane, which in turn is attached to a pleural layer lining the inner walls of the thorax, pericardium, and diaphragm. The area between these layers, called the pleural cavity, contains a thin film of fluid that allows the lung to slide easily during breathing.

The upper portion of the lung tapers upward to conform to the narrow shape of the rib cage, and extends into the neck about an inch above the level of the first rib. The base of the lung rests upon the surface of the diaphragm (see Fig. 1-13). The lungs occupy most of the space within the thoracic cavity except for the large area occupied by the pericardium. The lungs occupy not only the area between the ribs in front but also the deep concavity on either side of the spine. This space is formed by the rounded shape of the ribs, which extend outward from the sides of the spine and which also curve backward to the level of the spinous processes of the vertebrae before rounding forward to form the rib cage. The area from the top of the lungs down to the level of the heart constitutes roughly a third of the total area of the lung; at the level of the upper lung, this area is nearly one-half.

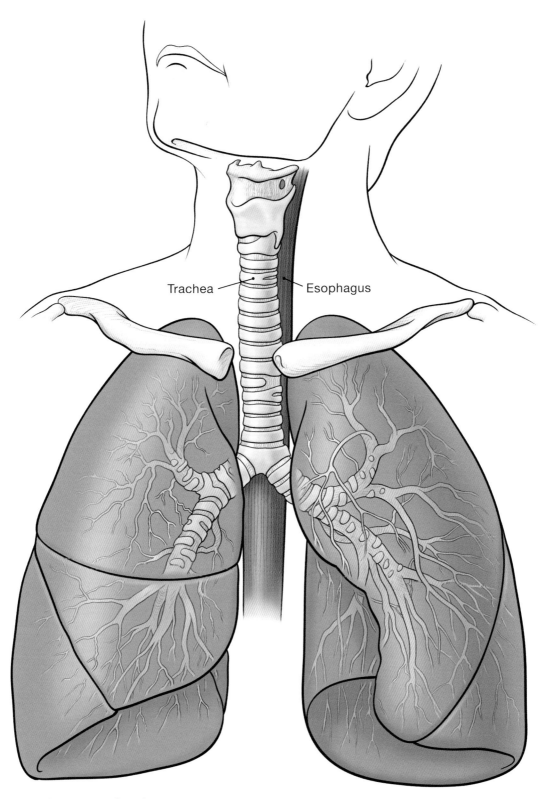

Trachea   Esophagus

Figure 1-28. The lungs and trachea.

Lung Capacity

The maximum amount of breath that can be taken into the lungs is about six or seven quarts or liters (this is the "total lung capacity"); after a forced exhalation, about two quarts remain (this is the "residual volume"). The difference between these two is the "vital capacity"—about four or five quarts or liters (Fig. 1-29a).

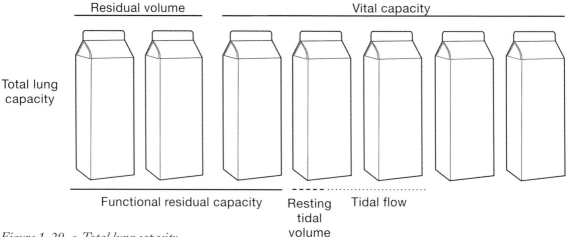

Figure 1-29. a. Total lung capacity.

Lung volume when the ribs and diaphragm are in a relaxed state (that is, when we are neither inhaling nor forcing air out of the lungs) is about three quarts; this is called the "functional residual capacity." During normal resting breathing, only about a pint, or half a liter, of air is inhaled above and beyond the functional residual capacity, and during shallow breathing even less; this is the "resting tidal volume" (Fig. 1-29b). During strenuous or forced exertion, the airflow is closer to two quarts—about three pints more than during quiet breathing. The air flowing into and out of the lungs—that is, the air that is actually being breathed—is the "tidal flow," as distinct from the three quarts or so of residual air always remaining in the lungs.

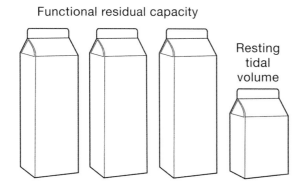

Figure 1-29. b. Lung capacity in relaxed state.

*T*he larynx, or organ of voice, is highly specialized and complex, but before examining its intricate anatomy, let's look at its basic design and function. In simple terms, the larynx is a valve located at the top of the trachea. This valve is composed of two muscles, or folds of muscle, that can be pulled apart or brought together. When we breathe normally, the two muscle folds are drawn apart, opening the valve so that air can pass through (Fig. 2-1a); when we swallow food or hold our breath, the muscle folds are tightened and drawn together, closing the valve so that food and water cannot enter the airway (Fig. 2-1b).

The valve also has a third function. When we want to produce sound, the muscle folds are drawn together—not as tightly as when we swallow, but loosely enough that they are free to vibrate as exhaled air passes between them. When this happens, they are set into motion by the airflow and begin to oscillate, generating sound waves that resonate in the space above the larynx, creating the fully formed sound of the human voice (Fig. 2-1c).

The larynx, then, is basically a vibration mechanism. It contains the oscillators that produce sound (the vocal folds), and it can bring them together so that they will vibrate when air (which is the power source) passes between them, and draw them apart during normal breathing. It can also tense and stretch the vocal folds in various ways in order to alter the volume, pitch, and types of vibration that occur.

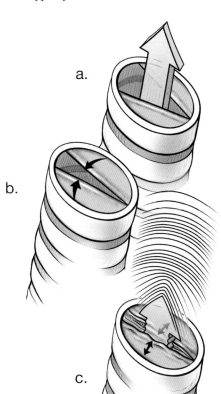

Figure 2-1. a. Vocal folds open.
b. Vocal folds closed.
c. Vocal folds approximated
for phonation.

Basic Structure of the Larynx

The larynx is mainly composed of four cartilages that form the housing for the vocal folds. At the top of the trachea is a ring-like cartilage similar to the rings of the trachea, called the cricoid cartilage. Above that is the thyroid cartilage, which is made up of two plates or wings that join in the front. Sitting on the back part of the cricoid cartilage within the wings or walls of the thyroid cartilage are two pyramid-shaped cartilages called the arytenoid cartilages (Fig. 2-2).

The vocal folds—the valve muscles that come together and vibrate when air hits them to create sound—are suspended between the two arytenoid cartilages and the inner front walls of the thyroid cartilage. When the arytenoid cartilages rotate inward, this brings the vocal folds together so that they vibrate as the air passing out of the lungs forces them open; when the arytenoid cartilages rotate back, the vocal folds are separated to allow air to pass through freely again (Fig. 2-2).

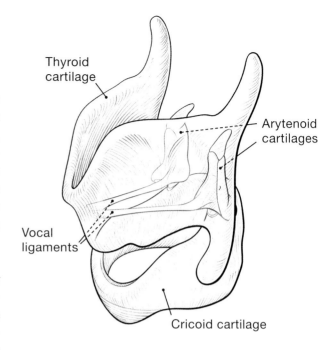

Figure 2-2. Cartilages and vocal cords.

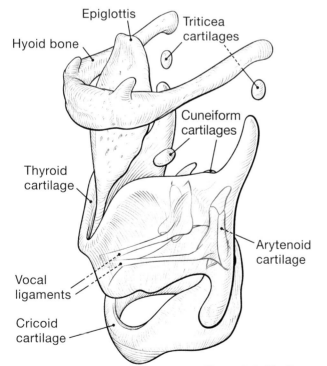

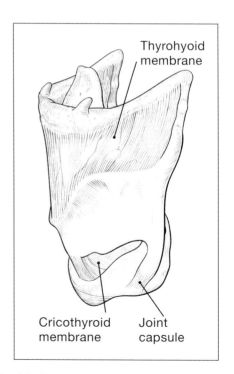

Figure 2-3. The framework of the larynx.

The Framework of the Larynx

The hyoid bone, the thyroid, cricoid, and arytenoid cartilages, the epiglottis, and the tiny corniculate and cuneiform cartilages form the complete framework of the larynx (Fig. 2-3). The thyroid cartilage is the most prominent part of the larynx (Fig. 2-4). Where the two plates of the thyroid join in front, they angle sharply forward in men, forming the prominent bump called the Adam's apple. The sides of the plates, or lamina, are rather smooth except toward the back, where a ridge, beginning at a tubercle or protrusion, runs down and forward to the lower border of the lamina, forming the oblique line. At the back part of each lamina there is a long upward projection called the superior cornu. Just above the thyroid cartilage is the U-shaped hyoid bone. This bone, which forms the root of the tongue, is an important part of the framework of the larynx because the larynx is suspended from the hyoid bone by a ligament attaching to the superior comu, as well as by the thyrohyoid membrane. A downward projection from the back part of the lamina, called the inferior cornu, forms a pivot with the sides of the cricoid cartilage (Fig. 2-4).

The cricoid, or ring, cartilage was given this name because of its resemblance to a signet ring—a ring with a large flat surface for imprinting one's seal. The front of the cricoid is narrow, not much thicker than the rings of the trachea below it; the back is thicker because it serves as attachment for the muscles that abduct, or open, the vocal folds, and as a surface area for the arytenoid cartilages (Fig. 2-4).

The arytenoid cartilages, when placed together, resemble a pitcher; hence their name (from the Greek word for pitcher). Because of their shape, the arytenoids are also sometimes called the "pyramid cartilages." At its base, the arytenoid forms a joint where it sits on the cricoid cartilage; there are also two protrusions or angles, the muscular process and the vocal process. The muscular process projects outward and backward and serves as attachment for the posterior and lateral cricoarytenoid muscles; the vocal process projects anteriorly and serves as attachment for the vocal folds (Fig. 2-4).

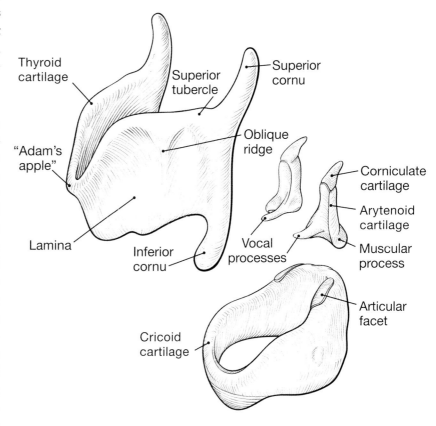

Figure 2-4. Thyroid, cricoid, and arytenoid cartilages.

The Epiglottis

The epiglottis is a broad, leaf-shaped cartilage situated at the front part of the larynx (Figs. 2-3 and 2-9). It stands upright and flaps down during swallowing to help to direct food toward the esophagus. It is attached at its base to the thyroid cartilage. Its sides angle backward and down to the arytenoid cartilages to form a kind of collar around the opening of the larynx called the aryepiglottic folds. The top of the arytenoid cartilage is not pointed but flat; the corniculate cartilages (or cartilages of Santorini) are small conical structures that extend the summit of the arytenoids and serve as attachment for the aryepiglottic folds (see Figs. 2-4 and 2-9). (The aryepiglottic folds themselves are stiffened by the cuneiform cartilages, also called the cartilages of Wrisberg, which are small, elongated cartilages embedded in the aryepiglottic folds.) This collar helps to keep food out of the larynx; with the wing of the thyroid cartilage on the other side, it forms a channel, called the piriform sinus, which allows liquids to pass around the larynx and into the esophagus (see Fig. 6-5).

This completes the basic framework of the larynx. The thyroid and cricoid cartilages and the base of the arytenoids are composed of a tough hyaline cartilage that tends to ossify with age; in contrast, the apices of the arytenoids, the epiglottis, the corniculate, and the cuneiform cartilages remain elastic.

Cricoarytenoid Joint

The cricoarytenoid joint, which is formed by the articulation of the arytenoid cartilages with the cricoid cartilage, is the key joint that makes it possible to open and close the vocal folds. On the back of the cricoid cartilage is a small notch; to either side of this notch, sloping down sharply and angling apart at 90 degrees to one another, are two elliptical, convex facets for articulation with the arytenoid cartilages (Fig. 2-5a). The base of the arytenoid cartilage is concave and sits nicely on these convex facets, forming a synovial joint that is surrounded by a joint capsule and reinforced by the posterior cricoarytenoid ligament (Fig. 2-5b).

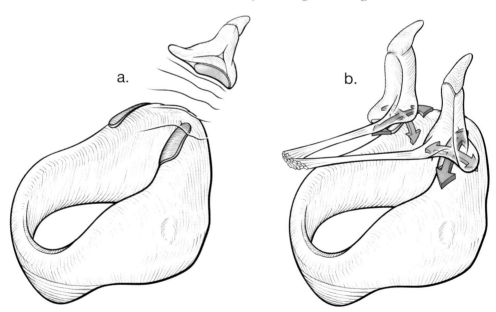

Figure 2-5. Cricoarytenoid joint: a. Articular facets on cricoid; b. Movement of arytenoid cartilages on the cricoid cartilage.

The posterior cricoarytenoid ligament arises from the cricoid cartilage and, fanning upward and obliquely forward, attaches to the medial surface of the arytenoid cartilage midway between the vocal process and the muscular process (not pictured).

The arytenoid cartilages move on the cricoid cartilages in two ways: inward and outward rocking, and medial and lateral sliding. The vocal processes come together when the arytenoid cartilages rock downward and inward, and apart when they rock upward and outward. When the cartilages slide toward the back, this brings the apices together but not the vocal processes (Fig. 2-5b).

Cricothyroid Joint

The other main joint of the larynx is the cricothyroid, which makes it possible to move the thyroid cartilage in relation to the cricoid cartilage. We saw a moment ago that the inferior cornua pivot on the cricoid cartilage. On the sides of the cricoid cartilage toward the back is a small raised facet; this articulates with a small facet on the inner surface of the inferior cornu (Fig. 2-6). This synovial joint is bounded by three ligaments. The posterior ceratocricoid ligament attaches toward the upper sides of the cricoid plate and runs downward and outward to attach to the inferior cornu of the thyroid. The lateral ceratocricoid ligament connects the inferior cornu with the side of the cricoid cartilage. Finally, the entire articulation is enclosed within a capsular ligament lined with a synovial membrane that lubricates the joint (see inset, Fig. 2-3).

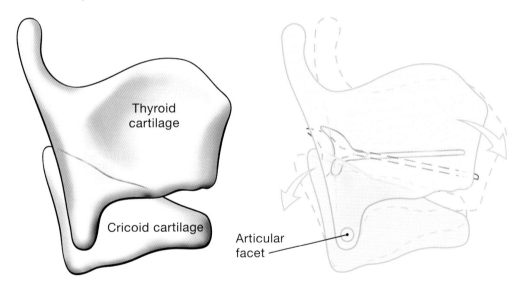

Figure 2-6. Cricothyroid joint.

Two movements take place at this joint: a rocking or pivoting of the thyroid cartilage in relation to the cricoid; and the thyroid can glide forward out of its articulation to move forward in relation to the cricoid cartilage. These actions, as we'll see later, stretch the vocal folds during vocalization and raise the pitch (Fig. 2-6; see also Fig. 2-18).

Conus Elasticus

Sometimes called the cricothyroid membrane, the conus elasticus is an elastic membrane connecting the upper border of the cricoid cartilage with the vocal folds and the front of the thyroid (Fig. 2-7). It is cone-shaped (hence its name), and attaches from the entire circumference of the cricoid cartilage and converges upward to join the front and back parts of the thyroid and the inner margins of the vocal folds—a kind of tent-like structure whose base is the cricoid cartilage and whose apex is the front of the thyroid. The part of the conus elasticus that connects the upper border of the front of the cricoid with the lower border of the front of the thyroid is sometimes called the cricothyroid ligament, or middle portion of the cricothyroid membrane. This central portion of the conus elasticus is thicker than the lateral portions. The lateral portions extend from the superior border of the cricoid cartilage to the margin of the vocal folds, forming a membrane from the top of the trachea to the vocal folds. This membrane provides a kind of lining for the vocal folds and so is continuous with the ligamentous bands or vocal ligaments.

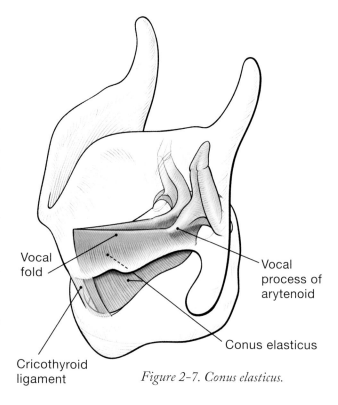

Figure 2-7. Conus elasticus.

The Interior of the Larynx

The cavity of the larynx extends from the superior aperture of the larynx to the cricoid cartilage (Fig. 2-8). Viewed in coronal section, the epiglottis is the large flap of tissue giving access to the larynx. The part of the cavity lying above the vocal folds is called the vestibule. The superior aperture of the larynx, or opening to the larynx from above, is bounded by the epiglottis in front, the arytenoids in back, and the aryepiglottic folds along the sides.

The vocal folds—sometimes referred to as the vocal cords—are actually part of a larger complex of muscles with two bellies or folds, an upper and a lower pair, sometimes called the superior and inferior thyroarytenoids (Fig. 2-8). The superior thyroarytenoids attach to the front of the thyroid cartilage just below the base of the epiglottis, and behind to the anterior surface of the arytenoid cartilages. They do not extend inward as far as the lower folds, are not actually involved in phonation, and are therefore sometimes called the false cords; they are more commonly known as the ventricular bands. Their main function is to assist the true cords in closing the valve tightly. Because they angle downward, they are designed to resist strong air pressure from below and are therefore well suited to closing up the airway (see Fig. 6-6).

The lower pair, or inferior thyroarytenoids, are the true vocal cords or folds and have come to be known as the vocalis muscle. The inner margin of each fold, as we will see in a moment, forms the vocal ligament. In contrast to the pink membrane of the vocal folds themselves, the ligaments are white in color. These ligaments are sometimes referred to as the vocal bands, in contrast to the vocal lips of the folds themselves. The vocalis muscles are very well suited to receive the flow of air from the lungs and to vibrate efficiently.

Because the vocalis muscle, when viewed from above, lies closer to the midline than the superior thyro-arytenoid, it is sometimes called "thyroarytenoid internus" and the superior thyroarytenoid (which lies to the outside) "thyroarytenoid externus." The generally accepted terminology now is simply vocalis for the inferior, true vocal folds and thyroarytenoid for the upper folds.

Between the thyroarytenoid and vocalis muscles is the ventricle of the larynx, which is an oblong cavity (Fig. 2-8). This sinus also has small air sacs that in some species fill with air. The ventricle of the larynx extends upward to form a small pouch or cavity between the superior or false vocal cord and the inner surface of the thyroid cartilage, called the sacculus laryngis, or laryngeal pouch. This sac contains mucus-producing glands and is surrounded by the aryepiglottic muscles

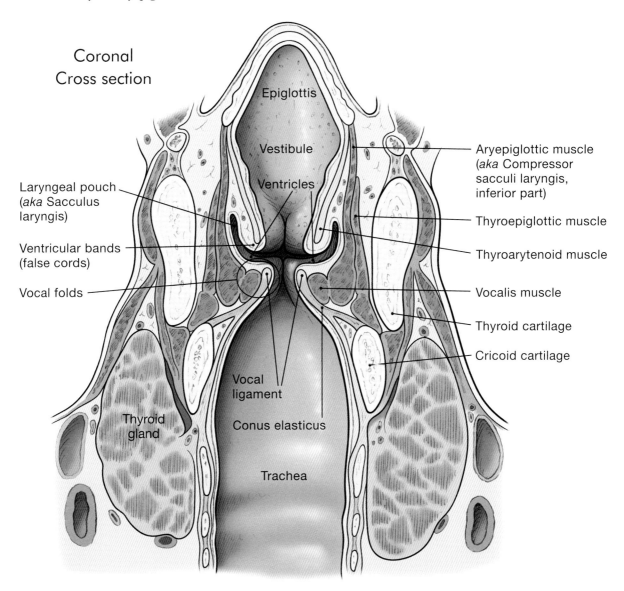

Figure 2-8. The interior of the larynx.

Muscles of the Epiglottis

The aryepiglottic muscle arises from the apex and anterior surface of the arytenoid cartilage and passes obliquely upward to join the aryepiglottic folds along the sides of the epiglottis (Fig. 2-9). This muscle is sometimes described in two parts, a superior arytenoepiglottideus muscle arising from the apex and anterior surface of the arytenoid cartilage and blending into the aryepiglottic folds, and an inferior arytenoepiglottideus muscle arising from the anterior surface of the arytenoid cartilage and blending into the anterior surface of the epiglottis. The superior portion of this muscle constricts the superior aperture of the larynx to prevent food from entering the airway during swallowing. The inferior portion of this muscle, sometimes called the compressor sacculi laryngis, compresses the sacculus; by squeezing the mucous glands, these muscles help to lubricate the vocal folds.

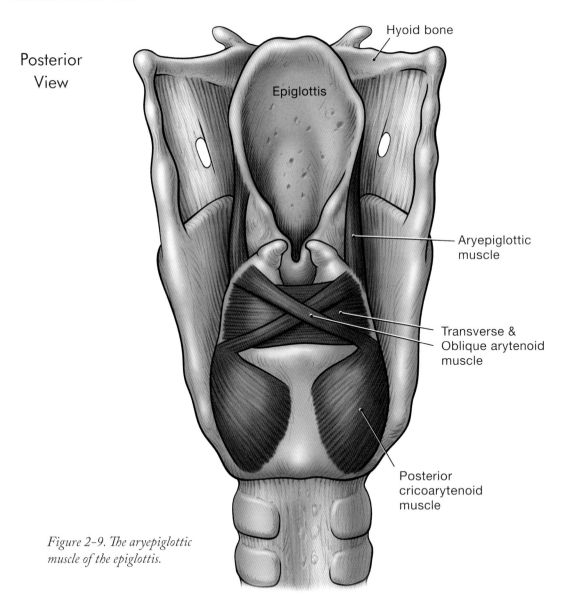

Posterior
View

Hyoid bone

Epiglottis

Aryepiglottic
muscle

Transverse &
Oblique arytenoid
muscle

Posterior
cricoarytenoid
muscle

Figure 2-9. The aryepiglottic muscle of the epiglottis.

The thyroepiglottic (or thyroepiglottideus) muscle arises from the inner surface of the thyroid cartilage just outside the thyroarytenoid muscle. Its fibers form the outer wall of the sacculus laryngis and also join into the aryepiglottic folds (Fig. 2-10). This muscle is a depressor of the epiglottis but also assists the aryepiglottic muscles in compressing the sacculus laryngis.

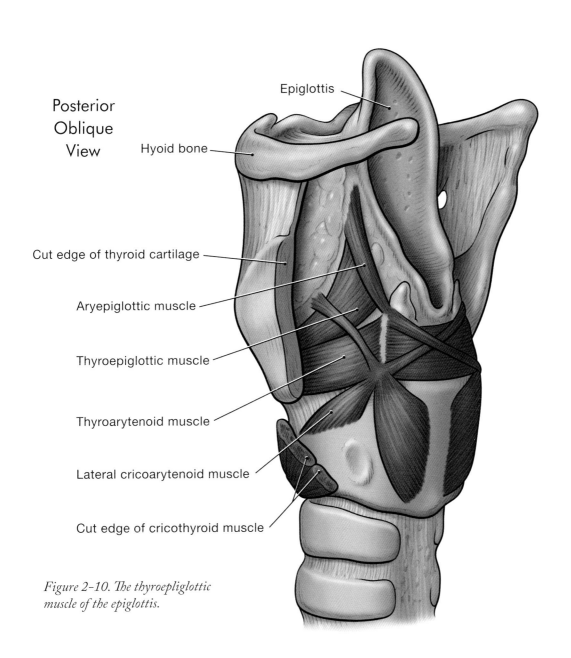

Posterior
Oblique
View

Epiglottis

Hyoid bone

Cut edge of thyroid cartilage

Aryepiglottic muscle

Thyroepiglottic muscle

Thyroarytenoid muscle

Lateral cricoarytenoid muscle

Cut edge of cricothyroid muscle

Figure 2–10. The thyroepiglottic muscle of the epiglottis.

The Structure of the Vocal Folds

The vocal folds are an exceedingly complex muscle whose structure is not yet fully understood. It is generally agreed that its main fibers are longitudinal, and run the length of the visible muscle. In the 1950s, some researchers claimed that none of its fibers ran the length of the muscle and that some originated at the arytenoids and attached into the vocal ligament (aryvocalis muscle) while others originated at the thyroid and attached into the vocal ligament (thyrovocalis muscle), creating a kind of diagonal pattern. When the muscles contracted, they would actually pluck the vocal ligament, so that the vibratory action of the vocal folds was not aerodynamic and myoelastic but actuated by nervous impulses. This view (called the "neurotaxic" or "neurochronaxic" theory) has been rejected, but the terminology corresponding to the two muscles sometimes persists (aryvocalis and thyrovocalis). Also, it is known that the folds contain some muscle fibers that run across the main direction of the longitudinal fibers; these may play a role in squeezing or thinning the vocal folds. In any case, the vocal folds have very delicate fibers and are able to contract in subtle ways, so that these fibers play a role in finely tuning the thickness of the vocal folds and controlling their vibrations.

Viewed under a microscope, the vocal folds consist of five layers: the epithelium; the superficial, intermediate, and deep layers of *lamina propria;* and the body of the vocalis muscle itself. The epithelium forms the outer mucosal layer and helps to keep the vocal folds lubricated; the next four layers become progressively firmer and provide both stiffness and elasticity to the vocal folds.

These five layers can be divided functionally into three groups. The epithelium and first layer of lamina propria form a loose mucosal structure that is well suited to vibrating when air flows through the glottis. The two deeper layers of lamina propria are composed of more tightly woven collagen fibers, which form the vocal ligament. The mucosal layer vibrates freely over the vocal ligament in singing. Underneath the mucosal layer and vocal ligament is the muscle itself, which is quite firm and can become even firmer when it contracts.

Intrinsic Muscles of the Larynx

There are five intrinsic muscles of the larynx. The first of these, the cricothyroid, moves the thyroid cartilage in relation to the cricoid. Because it lies on the outside of the thyroid and is supplied by the same nerves that supply the extrinsic muscles of the larynx, it is arguably an extrinsic, not an intrinsic, muscle of the larynx. The cricothyroid is a two-part muscle. The first part, called the oblique part or pars obliqua, arises from the side of the cricoid toward its front and, passing upward and backward, inserts into the inferior cornu and lower border of the lamina of the thyroid cartilage. The second part, called the vertical part or pars recta, inserts in the cricoid cartilage just in front of the oblique part and, passing more vertically upward, inserts into the lower border of the lamina of the thyroid (Fig. 2-11).

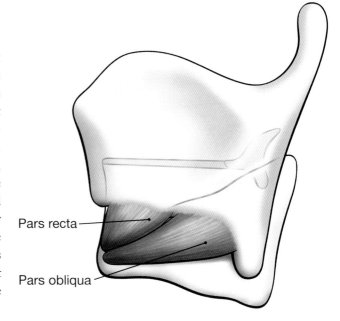

Pars recta

Pars obliqua

Figure 2-11. Cricothyroid muscle.

The Intrinsic Muscles of the Larynx

Five sets of muscles control the movement and action of the vocal folds, depicted in this drawing as colored bungee cords:

a. the posterior cricoarytenoid muscles open or abduct the glottis (red bungee cords);

b. the transverse arytenoid muscles close or adduct the glottis (blue bungee cord);

c. the lateral cricoarytenoid muscles close and partially adduct the glottis (purple bungee cords);

d. the cricothyroid muscles lengthen the vocal folds (yellow and orange bungee cords);

e. the thyroarytenoid muscles shorten or tense the vocal fold (green bungee cords)

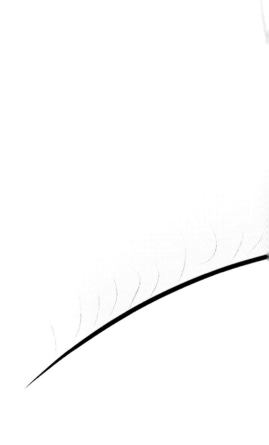

The vocalis muscle originates at the inner front surface of the thyroid cartilage to either side of the thyroid angle, and inserts into the vocal process of the arytenoid cartilage (Fig. 2-12). The innermost margin of the vocalis muscle, as we have seen, is made up of a ligament that is continuous with the conus elasticus. The ligament attaches to the tip of the vocal process; the vocalis muscle itself attaches to the tip just beside the vocal ligament and laterally to the anterior surface of the vocal process (see Figs. 2-7 and 2-8).

The thyroarytenoid muscle originates at the angle of the thyroid cartilage on its upper border and, pointing slightly outward, inserts broadly into the arytenoid cartilage from the vocal process to the muscular process. It is placed laterally to the fibers of the vocalis muscle (Fig. 2-12).

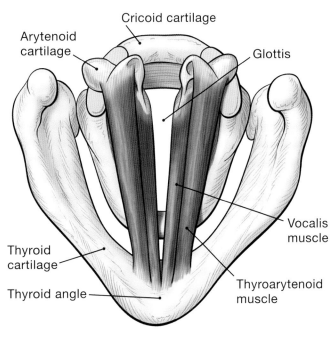

Figure 2-12. Vocalis and thyroarytenoid muscles, as viewed from above.

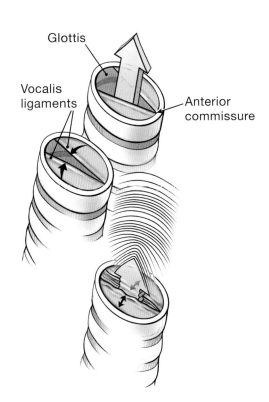

Figure 2-13. The glottis.

The glottis is the chink or aperture between the vocal folds. In men it averages 23mm in length, or just under an inch; in women, it averages 19mm in length, or about three-quarters of an inch. About three-fifths of this length, called the vocal portion, is the muscular part of the vocal fold; two-fifths is made up of the arytenoid cartilages and is called the respiratory portion. The glottis is changeable in shape, depending on whether the vocal folds are abducted or adducted; even when the folds themselves are closely approximated, as they are during phonation, there can still be a chink between the arytenoids. The acute angle of the glottis where the vocal folds attach to the thyroid cartilage is called the anterior commissure (Fig. 2-13).

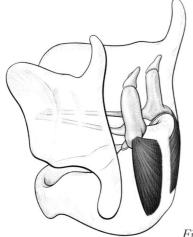

The posterior cricoarytenoid is the largest intrinsic muscle of the larynx. A prominent vertical ridge runs along the back plate of the cricoid; the muscle arises from the depressions on either side of this central ridge. Its fibers pass upward and outward to insert into the muscular process of the arytenoid cartilage, the upper fibers running nearly horizontally and the lower fibers passing almost vertically upward in order to converge into the same point on the arytenoid (Fig. 2-14).

Figure 2-14. The posterior cricoarytenoid muscle.

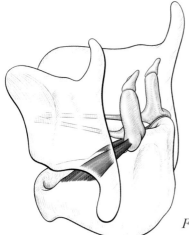

The lateral cricoarytenoid is situated at the sides of the cricoid cartilage. It arises from the external surface of the side of the cricoid cartilage and its upper border. Its fibers pass obliquely upward and backward and insert into the muscular process of the arytenoid cartilage (Fig. 2-15).

Figure 2-15. The lateral cricoarytenoid muscle.

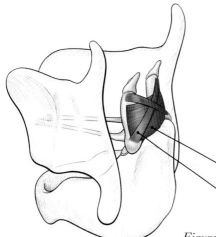

The transverse and oblique arytenoid muscles are situated at the back of the arytenoids and occupy the depressions at the back of each arytenoid. The transverse arytenoid arises from the outer border of the posterior surface of one arytenoid and attaches to the other. The oblique fibers pass from the base of one arytenoid to the apex of the other (Fig. 2-16).

Transverse arytenoid muscle

Oblique arytenoid muscle

Figure 2-16. The transverse and oblique arytenoid muscles.

Actions of the Intrinsic Muscles of the Larynx

The actions of the intrinsic muscles of the larynx can be divided into four categories:
• those that open the glottis by abducting the vocal folds (Figs. 2-17);
• those that close the glottis by adducting the vocal folds (Figs. 2-18, and 2-19);
• those that lengthen the vocal folds (Fig. 2-20);
• those that shorten and relax the vocal folds—the tensors (Fig. 2-21).

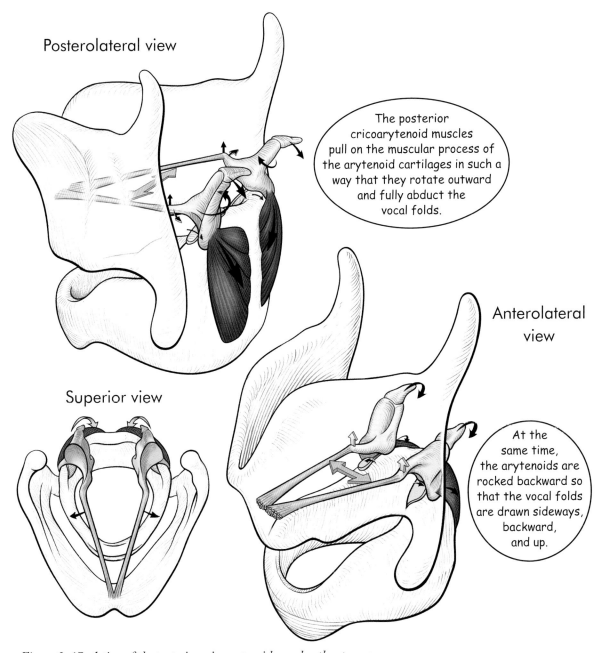

Figure 2-17. Action of the posterior cricoarytenoid muscles, the openers.

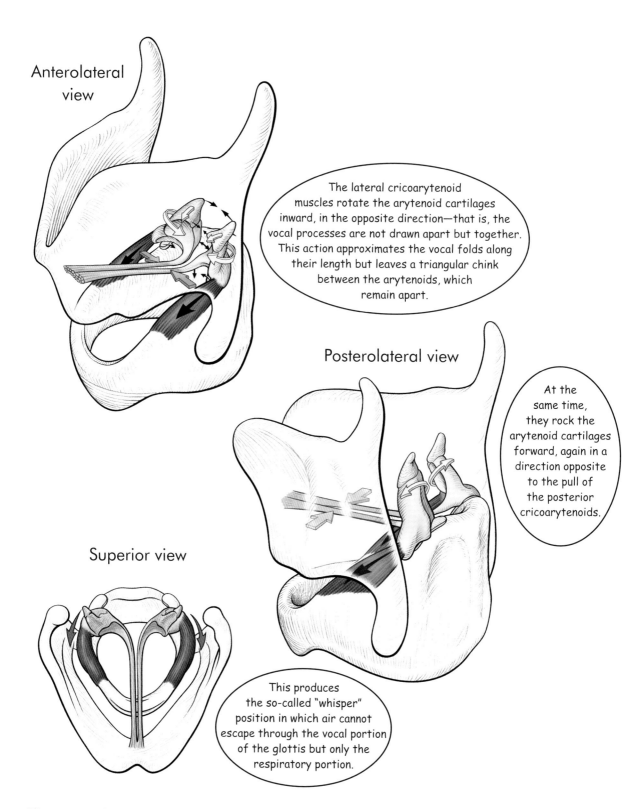

Anterolateral
view

The lateral cricoarytenoid
muscles rotate the arytenoid cartilages
inward, in the opposite direction—that is, the
vocal processes are not drawn apart but together.
This action approximates the vocal folds along
their length but leaves a triangular chink
between the arytenoids, which
remain apart.

Posterolateral view

At the
same time,
they rock the
arytenoid cartilages
forward, again in a
direction opposite
to the pull of
the posterior
cricoarytenoids.

Superior view

This produces
the so-called "whisper"
position in which air cannot
escape through the vocal portion
of the glottis but only the
respiratory portion.

Figure 2–18. Action of the lateral cricoarytenoid muscles, which close the glottis.

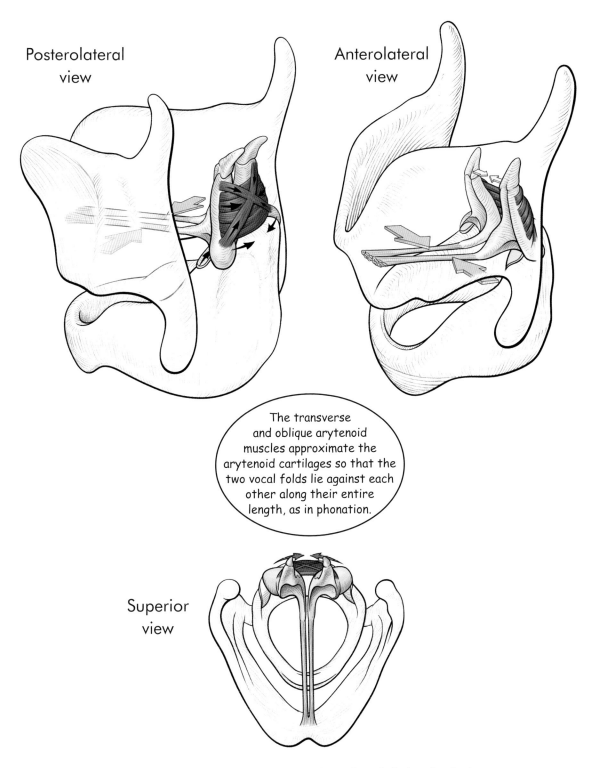

Posterolateral view

Anterolateral view

The transverse and oblique arytenoid muscles approximate the arytenoid cartilages so that the two vocal folds lie against each other along their entire length, as in phonation.

Superior view

Figure 2–19. Action of the transverse and oblique arytenoid muscles, which close the glottis.

The stretching of the vocal folds is performed by the cricothyroid muscle (Fig. 2-20), which attaches to the cricoid cartilage and the thyroid cartilage and pulls the two cartilages together in such a way that the distance between the two extremities of the vocal folds is increased, causing them to stretch. We saw above that the cricothyroid muscle has two parts: the vertical part (pars recta) and the oblique part (pars obliqua). The oblique part of the cricothyroid pulls the thyroid cartilage forward in relation to the cricoid (this is called translation); the vertical part pulls the thyroid cartilage down so that it pivots or rotates at the cricothyroid joint (Fig. 2-21). Acting together, the thyroid cartilage is rotated and pulled forward, which stretches the vocal folds by increasing the distance between their attachments at each end. If the thyroid cartilage is fixed by the extrinsic muscles, the cricoid cartilage will move in relation to the thyroid cartilage, rather than the other way around. In either case, however, the vocal folds are stretched.

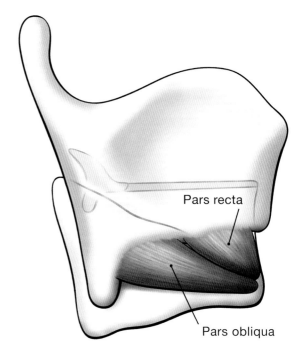

Figure 2-20. The cricothyroid, a stretching muscle.

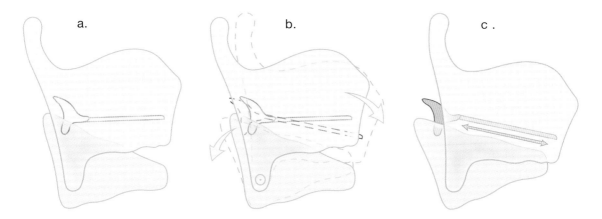

Figure 2-21. Stretching of the vocal folds.

The tensors are the thyroarytenoid and vocalis muscles (Fig. 2-22), which, by contracting, draw the arytenoid cartilages toward the thyroid cartilage and thus shorten (or relax) the vocal folds. The action of the vocalis and thyroarytenoid muscles thus regulates the elasticity and tension of the vocal folds, which also maintains closure of the glottis.

Acting together, the thyroarytenoid, the transverse arytenoid, and the aryepiglottic muscles tightly close the glottis; this occurs during swallowing and when we cough or hold our breath.

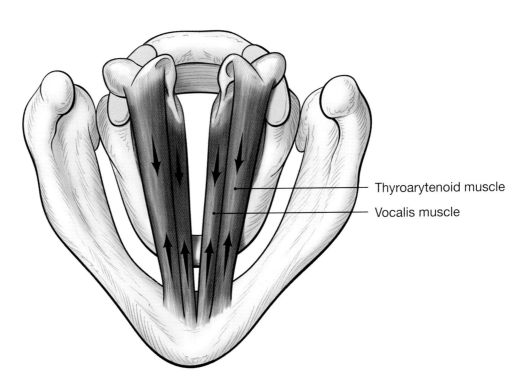

Thyroarytenoid muscle
Vocalis muscle

Figure 2-22. Tensors of the larynx.

Cricothyroid and Thyroarytenoid Antagonism

We saw earlier that the main stretcher of the vocal folds is the cricothyroid, which, by moving the thyroid and cricoid cartilage in relation to each other, draws the two opposite ends of the vocal folds apart, increasing their length. Opposed to this action are the vocalis and thyroarytenoid muscles, which pull the two poles together. In normal speaking or chest voice, the vocalis muscle must be active and requires the opposing stretching action of the cricothyroid to properly bring it into play.

Cricothyroid and Posterior Cricothyroid Antagonism

In order for the vocalis muscle to be stretched, the arytenoids must be anchored in place; otherwise, the force exerted by the tensors (vocalis) and stretchers (cricothyroid) would simply pull the arytenoid cartilages toward the front of the thyroid. This anchoring is accomplished by the posterior cricoarytenoids, which fix the arytenoids from behind.

Closure of the Glottis and Medial Compression

When the two ends of the vocal folds are drawn apart by the cricothyroid muscle, the vocal folds are stretched and become thinner. This causes them to gap in the middle so that they are imperfectly approximated even though the transverse arytenoids have approximated the arytenoid cartilages. The lateral cricoarytenoids are crucial in bringing about full closure of the glottis, exerting medial compression and in this way bringing the vocal cords together. The vocalis muscle must also be active, since no action of the arytenoids can totally ensure full approximation if the vocal folds themselves are entirely lax. Tension in the vocalis muscles pulls the vocal folds together, which in turn requires the antagonistic action of the posterior cricoarytenoids to anchor the arytenoids. So the transverse arytenoids are active in approximating the vocal folds; the lateral cricoarytenoids are active in increasing medial compression of the folds; the cricothyroids are active in stretching the vocal folds and opposing the pull of the vocalis muscle; the vocalis muscle is active in tensing the folds themselves; and the posterior cricoarytenoids anchor the arytenoid cartilages in place—a very active and synergistic coordination of muscles.

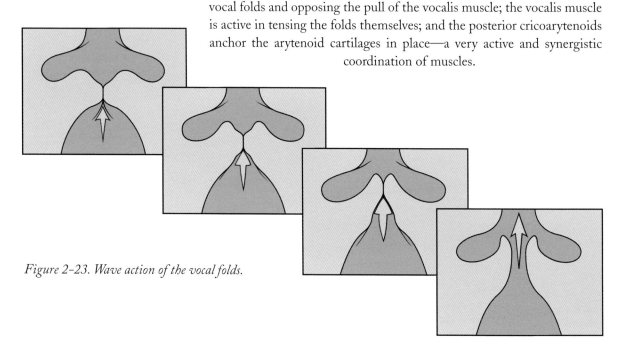

Figure 2-23. Wave action of the vocal folds.

Action of the Larynx Muscles in Chest Register

In chest voice, the transverse arytenoids are active in approximating the vocal folds, but only working lightly. The cricothyroids are active in regulating pitch, with increasing activity corresponding to higher pitch. The vocalis muscle acts antagonistically to the cricothyroid; by resisting the stretching effect of the cricothyroid, the vocalis remains thick, vibrating at a large amplitude and over its full surface with a wave-like motion that begins at the bottom and moves upward, creating the rich harmonics of the chest voice (Figs. 2-23 and 2-24). The activity of the vocalis also contributes to raising the pitch and to increasing its intensity. In order to anchor the arytenoids against these pulls, the posterior cricoarytenoid is active. The lateral cricoarytenoids are lightly active in bringing about medial compression of the vocal folds. Since the folds tend to gap under tension, and since the approximation of the transverse arytenoids does not bring the vocal processes together, the lateral cricoarytenoids are crucial in bringing about full closure of the glottis.

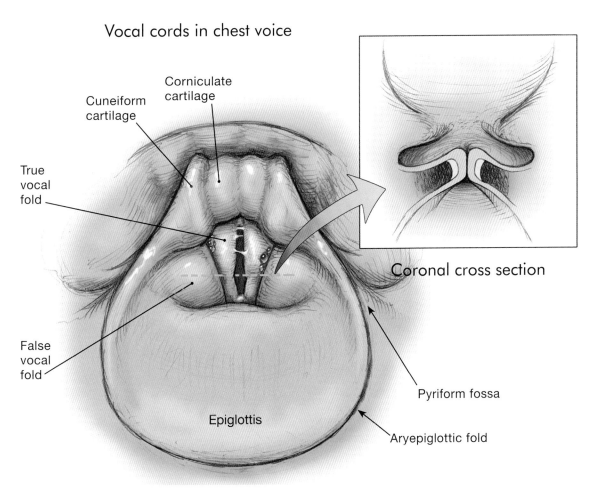

Figure 2-24. Vocal folds in chest voice: the vocal folds are relaxed and vibrate loosely, producing the rich chest voice. Inset: the entire body of each vocal fold is in contact with the other one as it vibrates.

Action of the Larynx Muscles in Falsetto Register

In falsetto register, the vocal folds are approximated by the transverse arytenoids. The cricothyroid is active only in the lower part of the falsetto range; at a certain point the vocal folds are maximally stretched and the cricothyroid activity simply remains at its maximum. The vocalis muscles are quite relaxed, allowing the cricothyroid, which is not being opposed by the tensing action of the vocalis muscle, to actively stretch the vocal folds (Fig. 2-25). Because the folds are stretched, they also become thinned and their amplitude increases; since the vocal folds are no longer vibrating with a wave-like motion and only the vocal bands are moving, this creates a thin falsetto sound. The vocalis muscle does contract somewhat to regulate the pitch, but much less than in chest voice. Against this pull, the posterior cricoarytenoids must be somewhat active in order to anchor the arytenoid cartilages. Because the vocal folds are stretched and thinned, they tend to gap a great deal in falsetto, preventing the glottis from closing entirely. In order to resist this gapping tendency, the lateral cricoarytenoids must actively work to maintain medial compression of the vocal folds. Also, because the vocal folds do not increase in length in the upper octaves of the falsetto, pitch is determined by longitudinal tension on the vocal ligaments, aided by the extrinsic musculature as well as breath pressure.

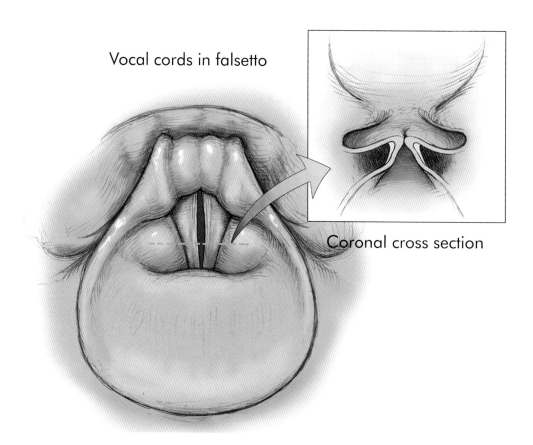

Vocal cords in falsetto

Coronal cross section

Figure 2-25. Vocal folds in falsetto: the vocal folds are taut and vibrate more quickly, producing the more flute-like falsetto sound. Inset: only the inner margin of each vocal fold is in contact as it vibrates.

Action of the Larynx Muscles in Head Register

Several elements of chest voice combine with falsetto register to produce the head voice. In order to produce the higher pitches of the head voice, the cricothyroid muscle must work actively to maintain full stretch on the vocal folds. To maintain the full tone of the head voice, however, the vocalis muscle contracts and continues to actively vibrate, as it does in chest voice. Because the vocal folds are active, they gap less than in falsetto and air is therefore utilized more efficiently, requiring less breath to produce the tone. Also, when the vocalis muscles are active, there is more glottal resistance and more aerodynamic efficiency. The transverse arytenoids must also be active in order to maintain approximation of the vocal folds and intensity of tone as well as efficiency of breath. Activity of the lateral cricothyroids is also high; this maintains medial compression of the glottis while the folds are under maximum lengthening and tension. Because the arytenoids must be anchored against these strong pulls, the posterior cricoarytenoids are also highly active in head voice. As with falsetto, the vocal folds are maximally stretched, so that rise in pitch is associated with an increase in longitudinal tension of the vocal bands. This, and the need to maintain full stretch on vocal ligaments with an active vocalis muscle, requires very active working of the extrinsic musculature.

CHAPTER 3

THE EXTRINSIC MUSCLES OF THE LARYNX

We've seen that the larynx and its intrinsic muscles precisely adjust the vocal folds so that they vibrate efficiently, creating subtle nuances in timbre, focus, and pitch. As a sound-producing mechanism, the larynx is the principal organ of voice. But the larynx is also suspended within a network of throat muscles that act on it from without and therefore form its extrinsic musculature.

The extrinsic muscles of the larynx serve two functions. First, they assist in swallowing. We saw in the last chapter that the primary function of the larynx is to close up the airway in order to prevent food from entering. To further protect the airway, extrinsic muscles attaching to the hyoid bone and larynx pull the larynx up and forward. This takes the larynx out of the path of the food and helps to close up the collar of the larynx, ensuring that the food passes into the esophagus and not the trachea (see sidebar on page 66).

The extrinsic muscles also play a crucial role in vocalization. To function efficiently as a sound-producing organ, the larynx must not be hindered in its action by muscular tension, and the throat, as the resonating chamber, must be open. When we sing, however, the swallowing muscles that elevate and constrict the larynx tend to come into play, particularly when we sing in falsetto or head registers. In order to maintain a low position of the larynx and an open throat, the action of the swallowing muscles that elevate the larynx must be countered by muscles pulling down on the larynx, antagonistically supporting it within a web of muscles. This makes it possible to raise the pitch without interfering with the vibratory action of the larynx, and to maintain an open throat. Engaging the suspensory muscles in this way is one of the most important skills a trained singer must learn.

The Suspensory Muscles of the Larynx

Four muscles directly form the suspension of the larynx during the act of singing. We saw earlier that the hyoid bone is located directly above the thyroid cartilage, which is suspended from the hyoid bone by the thyrohyoid ligament. Corresponding to the thyrohyoid ligament is the thyrohyoid muscle, which connects the thyroid cartilage directly above to the hyoid bone, supporting the larynx from above. The thyrohyoid muscle is a continuation of the sternothyroid muscle, originates at the oblique line of the thyroid cartilage just in front of the sternothyroid, and runs vertically upward to insert into the body and cornua of the hyoid bone (Fig. 3-1).

Another crucial elevator of the larynx is the stylopharyngeus muscle. On the temporal bones on the base of the skull are two small spikes called the styloid processes (Fig. 3-2). Stylopharyngeus arises from the base of the styloid processes and, angling forward, attaches to the posterior border of the thyroid cartilage and to either side of the walls of the pharynx, which we'll look at in Chapter Four. Stylopharyngeus directly connects the thyroid cartilage as well as the sides of the pharynx with the styloid process, pulling upward on the larynx and throat (Fig. 3-1).

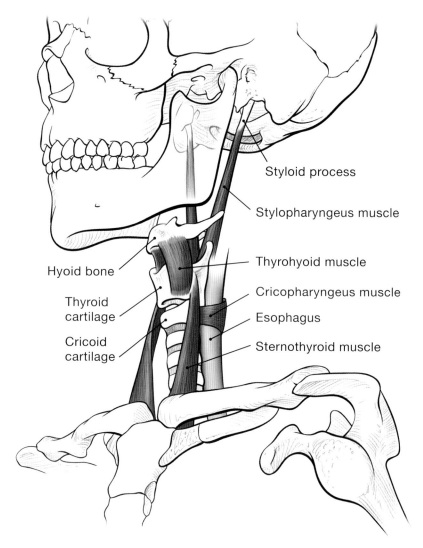

Figure 3-1. Suspensory muscles of the larynx.

Countering the upward force of these muscles is the sternothyroid, which originates at the inner border of the sternum and the first rib and inserts into the oblique ridge on the wing of the thyroid cartilage (Fig. 3-1).

Cricopharyngeus is another crucial suspensory muscle, anchoring the thyroid cartilage of the larynx directly back to the pharynx and esophagus. This muscle originates at the cricoid cartilage and is continuous with the inferior constrictor of the pharynx (Fig. 3-1).

Based on the directions indicated, we can infer what actions are performed by these muscles. The thyrohyoid and stylopharyngeus, as well as palatopharyngeus (which we'll talk about later when we look at the palate), pull the larynx up and back; they are therefore elevators of the larynx. The sternothyroid muscle pulls the larynx down and is therefore a depressor; cricopharyngeus anchors it back and down and is therefore another depressor. So the larynx is suspended from the hyoid bone and connected back and up to the skull via stylopharyngeus; it is connected below to the sternum via sternothyroid; and it is connected behind to the esophagus via cricopharyngeus—a complex web of muscular support that extends up, back, and to the sternum below and to the throat directly behind, so that it is literally supported within a muscular scaffolding, sometimes called the "suspensory muscles" of the larynx, which antagonistically support it from various directions (Fig. 3-1).

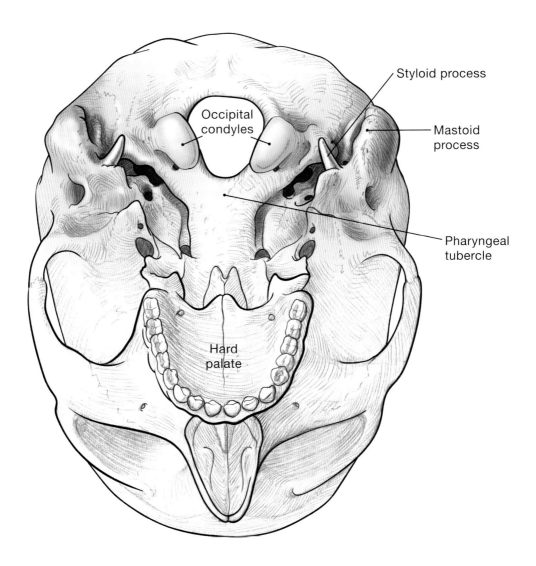

Figure 3-2. Base of skull with styloid and mastoid processes.

wo other muscles contribute indirectly to the suspensory support of the larynx during vocalization. Sternohyoid directly connects the hyoid bone with the sternum; it originates at the clavicle and sternum on its inside border and passes upward to insert into the lower border of the body of the hyoid bone (Fig. 3-3). It assists the sternothyroid in actively *pulling down* on the larynx and countering the upward pull of the elevators.

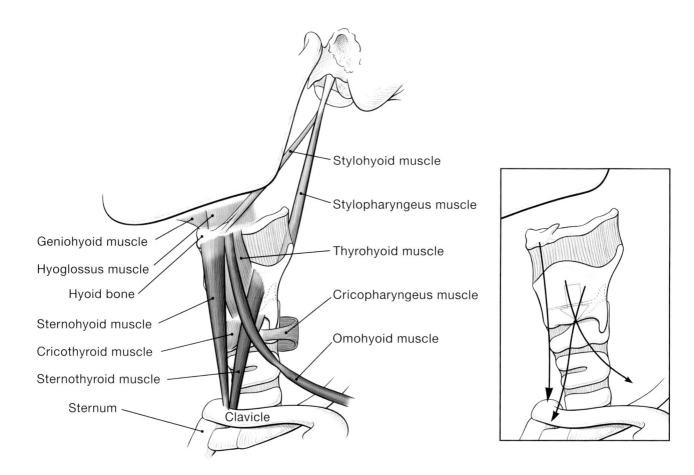

Geniohyoid muscle

Hyoglossus muscle

Hyoid bone

Sternohyoid muscle

Cricothyroid muscle

Sternothyroid muscle

Sternum

Clavicle

Stylohyoid muscle

Stylopharyngeus muscle

Thyrohyoid muscle

Cricopharyngeus muscle

Omohyoid muscle

Figure 3-3. Complete suspensory muscles of the larynx.

Omohyoid arises from the upper border of the scapula and, passing upward, changes angle to pass almost vertically upward to insert into the lower border of the body of the hyoid bone (Fig. 3-3). Where the muscle forms an angle, it is actually tendinous; this section is held in place by a sheath formed by the cervical fascia. Like sternohyoid and sternothyroid, it depresses or lowers the larynx.

Action of the Suspensory Muscles during Singing

The stabilizing action of the suspensory muscles aids in the production of high tones in specific ways. As we saw in the last chapter, the cricothyroid muscle raises the pitch by stretching the vocal folds. Activity of the cricothyroids, however, is associated with the constricting action of the throat muscles, so that untrained singers tend to tighten the larynx as they ascend in pitch. They also tend to raise the larynx because, as the pitch increases, the cricothyroids are at their maximal activity, and stretching of the vocal bands has to be aided by elevators of the larynx (such as thyrohyoid, stylohyoid, geniohyoid, and hyoglossus), which pull upward on the thyroid and tip it forward, stretching the cords (Fig. 3-4a). All of this activity is associated with tightening the throat, as can clearly be seen in untrained singers who "reach" for high notes by *raising the larynx* and tightening the entire neck and larynx in the process (Figs. 3-4b and c).

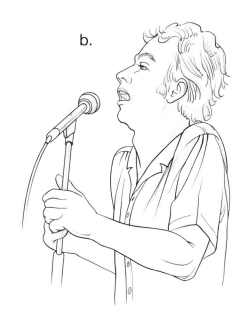

b.

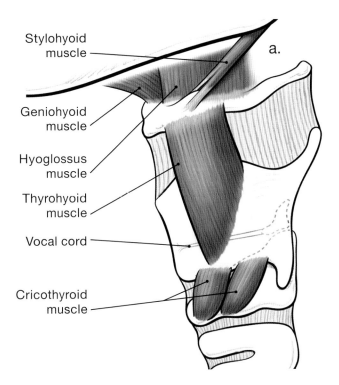

Stylohyoid muscle

a.

Geniohyoid muscle

Hyoglossus muscle

Thyrohyoid muscle

Vocal cord

Cricothyroid muscle

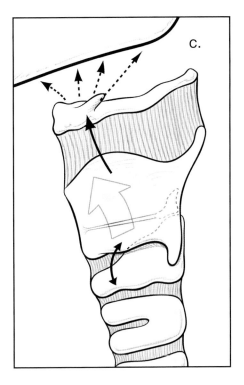

c.

Figure 3-4. a. Elevation of the larynx in singing; b. Strained appearance of singer; c. Lines of force of the elevators.

Trained singers, in contrast, are able to raise the pitch without elevating the larynx or tightening the throat. This is partly because they are more familiar and comfortable with the falsetto register, and therefore do not force the chest voice activity into the falsetto range. They are also able to engage the extrinsic muscles that depress the larynx in order to actively counter the upward pull of the extrinsic muscles that elevate the larynx—in particular, the sternothyroid and sternohyoid muscles (Fig. 3-5). Pulling down on the larynx and maintaining it in a lower position has two beneficial effects. First, it pulls the thyroid cartilage forward and in this way assists the cricothyroid in lengthening the vocal folds. Second, lowering the larynx maintains a more open and elongated throat.

The downward pull of the sternohyoid and sternothyroid muscles is assisted by the trachea, which exerts a "tracheal pull" on the cricoid cartilage, and the esophagus, which tends to pull downward on the arytenoid cartilages. This pulls the cricoid cartilage backward and anchors it, stretching the vocal folds to produce a high tone while maintaining a low position of the larynx.

Another elevator that actively participates in the antagonistic activity of the extrinsic muscles is the stylopharyngeus muscle. By pulling up on the horns of the thyroid cartilage, this muscle tilts the thyroid forward, assisting in the stretching action on the vocal folds (as in Fig. 3-5). And since the origins of the muscle at the styloid processes are farther apart than its insertions in the throat, the stylopharyngeus pulls the pharynx up and outward, helping to dilate or open the throat. Because the sternothyroid is antagonistically opposing the action of the elevators, the stylopharyngeus muscle can produce these effects without actually raising the larynx.

Activating the suspensory muscles that support the larynx in a balanced, antagonistic action has a marked effect on timbre, resonance, and vocal range. The ability of the larynx to function optimally, as well as the ability to sing with an "open throat," depend to a large extent upon the antagonistic action of the suspensory muscles of the larynx.

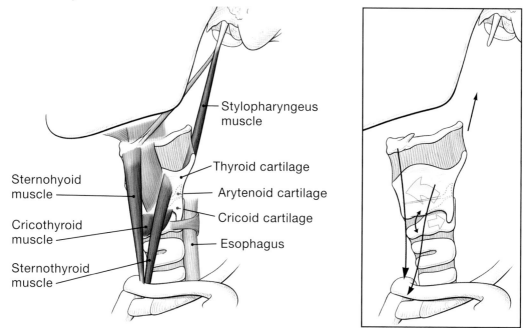

Figure 3-5. Action of the suspensory muscles during singing. Inset shows lines of force of the muscles.

Supported Falsetto

The extrinsic muscles are particularly important in producing the supported falsetto (Fig. 3-6). During normal falsetto voice, the vocalis muscle is relaxed, while the muscles that raise the pitch, the cricothyroid muscles, actively thin the vocal cords, countered by the posterior cricoarytenoid muscle. In the supported falsetto, the suspensory muscles more actively support the larynx. In particular, the sternothyroid muscle actively contributes to the stretching process, as well as the thyrohyoid, to help the closers oppose the action of the cricothyroid. This helps to reinforce the blend between registers because, instead of a break between registers, the antagonism is maintained throughout—a truly supported voice. Engaging the suspensory muscles in this way makes it possible to manage the register break skillfully and is a basic part of the singer's training.

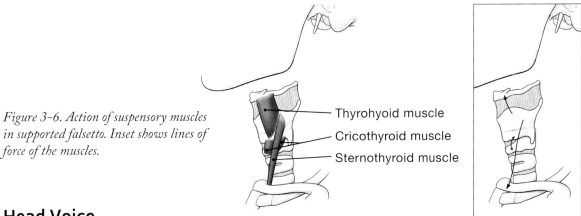

Figure 3-6. Action of suspensory muscles in supported falsetto. Inset shows lines of force of the muscles.

Thyrohyoid muscle
Cricothyroid muscle
Sternothyroid muscle

Head Voice

In "head" voice, the suspensory muscles of the larynx are at their highest activity (Fig. 3-7). In head voice the vocalis remains active and therefore opposes the cricothyroid. The cricothyroid is at its maximum activity and cannot lengthen the vocal folds beyond a certain point; it is actively assisted by the stylopharyngeus and palatopharyngeus (see Fig. 4-6) muscles, which pull up on the thyroid and, in conjunction with the sternothyroid, tilt the thyroid cartilage forward and down. These upward pulls are countered by the sternothyroid, sternohyoid, and omohyoid muscles, which oppose the upward pull of the elevators. Finally, the cricopharyngeus muscle actively anchors the cricoid cartilage behind, enabling the thyroid cartilage to move freely on the cricoid cartilage and to produce full stretching of the vocal folds. Because the larynx has not been raised or tightened, it is free to vibrate, and because it is low and the pharynx is fully open, it is able to produce the powerful resonances of the head voice.

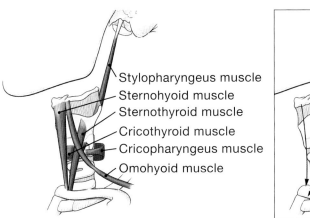
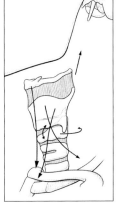

Stylopharyngeus muscle
Sternohyoid muscle
Sternothyroid muscle
Cricothyroid muscle
Cricopharyngeus muscle
Omohyoid muscle

Figure 3-7. Action of suspensory muscles in head voice. Inset shows lines of force of the muscles.

The Hyoid Apparatus

As the only bone in the region of the throat and the only free-floating bone in the body, the horseshoe-shaped hyoid is a central point of attachment for the muscles of the throat (Figs. 3-8 and 3-9). Because of the hyoid bone's shape, the Greeks named it after the letter upsilon. You can identify the hyoid bone if you pinch your throat with thumb and forefinger just above your larynx and swallow or wag your tongue; you will feel the hyoid bone and larynx move.

The central portion or body of the hyoid bone is thick; two horns project backward from the body and two smaller horns project inward and serve as attachments for the stylohyoid ligament. It is suspended from the styloid processes by the stylohyoid ligament and the stylohyoid muscle, which is the one remaining elevator of the hyoid we haven't yet looked at (Fig. 3-9). Stylohyoid arises from the base of the styloid process and, passing forward and downward, inserts into the body of the hyoid bone.

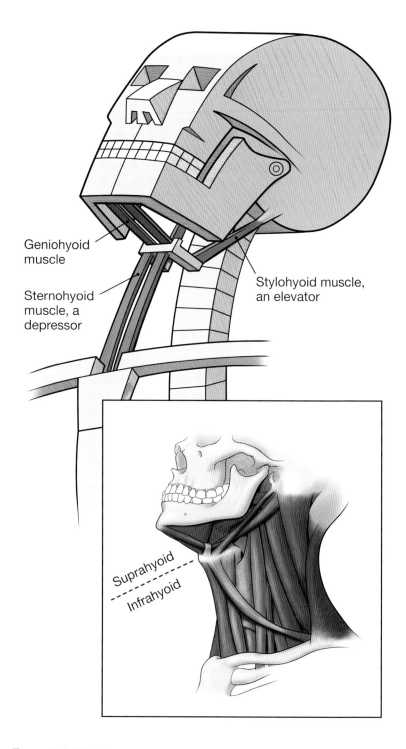

Geniohyoid muscle

Sternohyoid muscle, a depressor

Stylohyoid muscle, an elevator

Suprahyoid

Infrahyoid

Figure 3-8. Hyoid apparatus.

The hyoid bone serves three essential purposes. First, as we've already seen, it serves as an attachment for the larynx and for the muscles that elevate and lower the larynx in swallowing. Second, it is a key anchor point for the muscles on the floor of the mouth that depress or open the jaw. Third, it forms an anchor for the tongue and is for this reason sometimes referred to as the "tongue bone" (Fig. 3-8).

Because the hyoid bone is the central attachment of the network of throat muscles, the muscles of the throat are sometimes divided into those supporting and moving the larynx and hyoid bone from above, called the suprahyoid muscles, and those acting on the larynx and hyoid from below, called the infra-hyoid muscles. The suprahyoid muscles are mainly on the underside of the jaw and skull; they pull the hyoid bone and larynx up and forward and move the jaw (inset, Fig. 3-8).

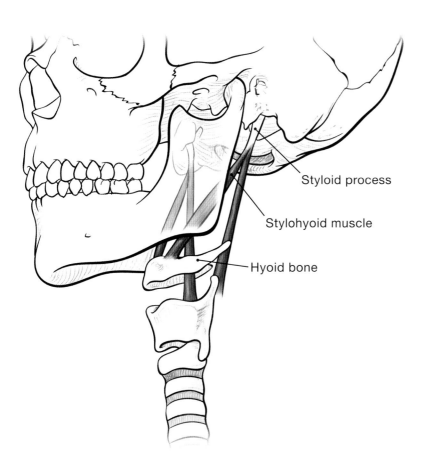

Styloid process

Stylohyoid muscle

Hyoid bone

THE HYOID BONE

The hyoid bone is the only bone in the throat region and serves three essential purposes.

• First, it serves as an attachment for the larynx and for the muscles that elevate and lower the larynx in swallowing.

• Second, it is a key anchor point for the muscles on the floor of the mouth that depress or open the jaw.

• Finally, it provides a stable base for the tongue (for this reason it is sometimes referred to as the "tongue bone").

Figure 3-9. Styloid process and hyoid bone.

Muscles of the Hyoid Bone and Jaw

We have now looked at several of the elevators and depressors of the hyoid bone and larynx. There are several more extrinsic muscles attaching to the hyoid bone on the underside of the jaw that form part of the extrinsic musculature of the larynx.

The digastric is a sling-like muscle that extends from the inner side of the lower jaw to the mastoid process on the base of the skull. It has two muscle bellies joined by a tendon that passes through a fibrous loop attaching to the sides of the hyoid bone (Fig. 3-11).

Styloglossus arises from the styloid processes and attaches to the sides of the tongue (Fig. 3-11).

Mylohyoid, a pair of flat and fan-shaped muscles, forms the floor of the mouth. Its fibers run at a downward angle from the inner surface of the symphysis and body of the jaw, joining along the midline at a tendinous band and, at its posterior end, to the hyoid bone (Fig. 3-10).

Geniohyoid lies just above mylohyoid and runs from the inner surface of the symphysis of the jaw to the hyoid bone (Fig. 3-10).

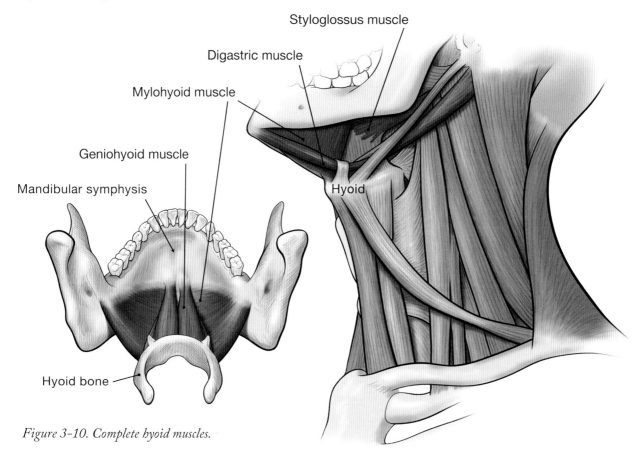

Figure 3-10. Complete hyoid muscles.

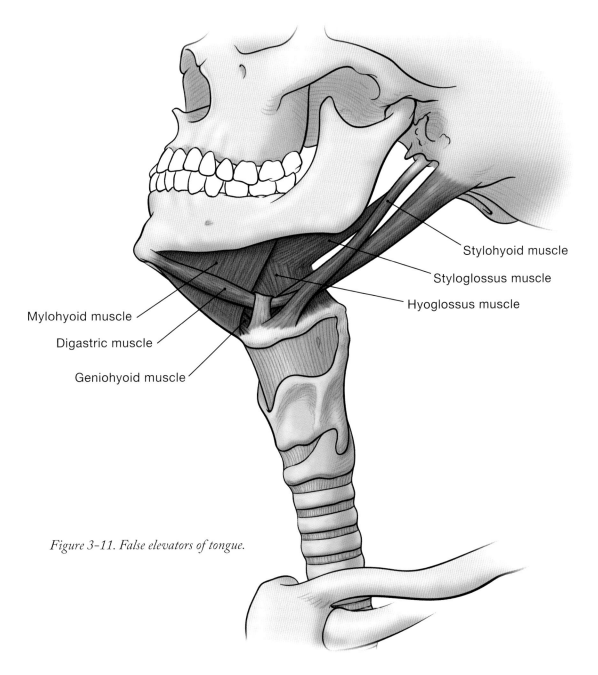

Mylohyoid muscle

Digastric muscle

Geniohyoid muscle

Stylohyoid muscle

Styloglossus muscle

Hyoglossus muscle

Figure 3-11. False elevators of tongue.

These muscles perform two critical functions. First, they depress or open the lower jaw; second, they elevate the hyoid bone and draw the hyoid bone and tongue forward during swallowing. Geniohyoid and mylohyoid are false elevators of the larynx; the tendency to overuse these muscles can often be detected in popular singers who appear to have a kind of double chin from overworking these muscles (Fig. 3-4). However, it is possible that the geniohyoid muscle, which pulls the hyoid bone forward in swallowing, may have a role in singing high notes. Because of the direction of its pull, its effect is to rotate the thyroid cartilage forward, which helps to stretch the vocal folds and thus assists the cricothyroid. The genioglossus may also assist in rotating the thyroid cartilage forward and widening the pharynx.

The infrahyoid muscles attach mainly to the sternum and depress or lower the hyoid bone and larynx. The thyrohyoid muscle is a continuation of the sternothyroid muscle and originates at the oblique line of the thyroid cartilage just in front of sternothyroid and runs vertically upward to insert into the body and cornua of the hyoid bone. These muscles, including the thyrohyoid, are collectively known as the "strap" muscles (Fig. 3-12).

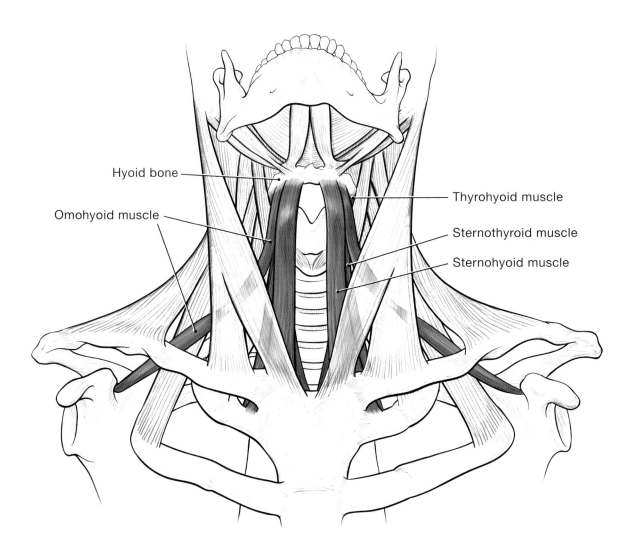

Figure 3–12. Sternohyoid, sternothyroid, thyrohyoid, and omohyoid are all depressors of the hyoid and larynx and are known collectively as the "strap" muscles.

*A*s the opening to the digestive tract, the mouth and pharynx, or throat, have an obvious and essential role in the processing of food. Food taken into the mouth is chewed by the movable jaw, positioned by the tongue, and drawn down the throat into the esophagus and stomach. The mouth and pharynx also double as an air passageway, which, as we've seen, require complex actions of the tongue, palate, and larynx to ensure that food does not go down the airway.

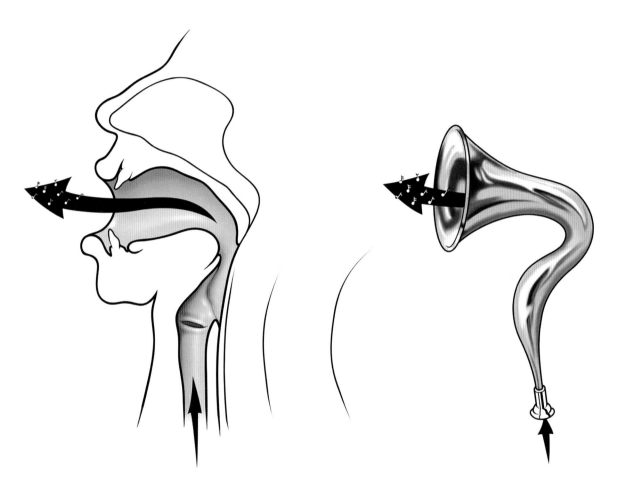

Figure 4–1. The vocal tract.

The mouth and pharynx also serve a crucial role in the production of sound and speech. Sounds produced by the larynx are shaped by the pharynx and mouth, which form the vocal tract, to create different vowel sounds, and chopped up by the lips, teeth, tongue, and palate to produce consonants, resulting in the distinct, articulated sounds of human speech (Fig. 4-1).

The mouth, or oral cavity, is separated from the nasal cavity by the hard palate, which forms the roof of the mouth. The mouth opens into the throat, or pharynx. The pharynx is roughly four and a half inches in length and extends from the base of the skull to the bottom of the larynx. The pharynx can be divided into three sections—the nasopharynx, oropharynx, and laryngopharynx (also known as the hypopharynx). The nasal section lies behind the nose and extends to the soft palate; the oral part extends from the soft palate to the epiglottis; the laryngeal section extends from the epiglottis to the cricoid cartilage, the lowest part of the larynx. At this point the common passageway for food and air splits into the trachea in front and the esophagus in back (Fig. 4-2).

The nasopharynx, which serves only for the passage of air, is not variable in shape. In contrast, the lower two-thirds of the pharynx can be constricted, dilated, and lengthened. These movements evolved first for the purpose of swallowing and breathing, but they also function as part of the vocal mechanism and play a critical role in the modulation of the voice.

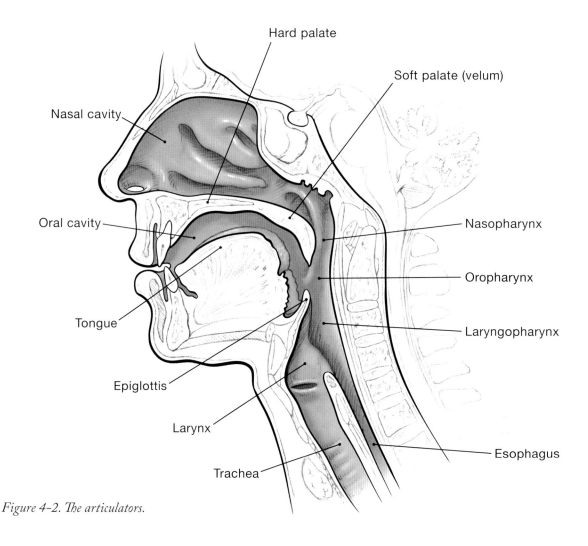

Figure 4-2. The articulators.

Muscles of the Mouth and Throat

The passageway of the throat is entered by the mouth, the opening of which is protected by orbicularis oris, the muscle forming the lips. Buccinator forms the muscular walls of the cheek (Fig. 4-3). It arises from the maxilla just above the molars and from the mandible just below the molars, and from the pterygomandibular raphe, a ligamentous band of tissue that also serves as the attachment for the superior constrictor. Its fibers run horizontally to blend continuously into the fibers of orbicularis oris. Its function is to compress the cheek to position food for chewing.

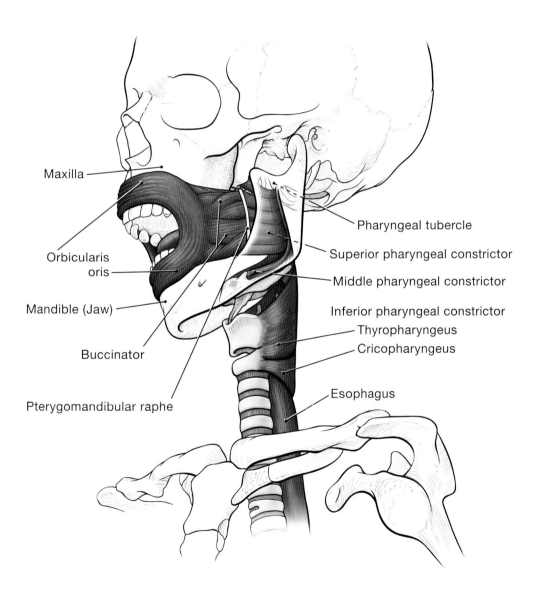

Figure 4-3. Muscles of the mouth and throat.

The constrictor muscles form the walls of the pharynx (Figs. 4-3 and 4-4). Originating on either side of the throat, these muscles wrap around to the back to form a seam along the midline of the back of the throat called the median pharyngeal raphe. This seam attaches above to the pharyngeal tubercle, a small bump on the base of the skull just in front of the foramen magnum (see Fig. 3-2); like the hyoid bone and larynx, the constrictors are suspended from the base of the skull.

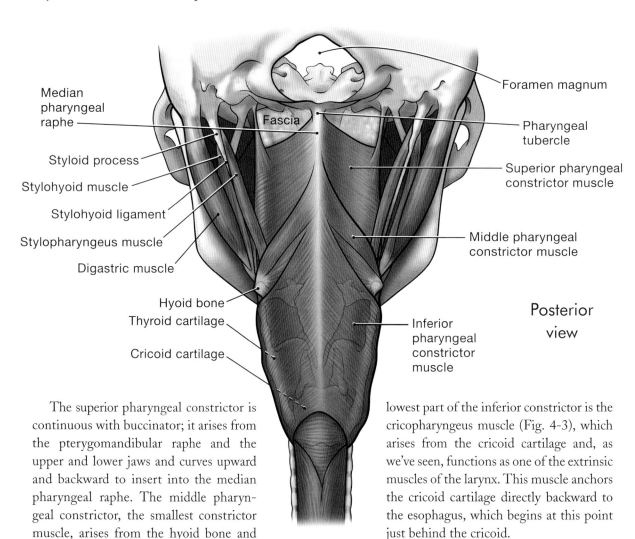

Median pharyngeal raphe

Styloid process

Stylohyoid muscle

Stylohyoid ligament

Stylopharyngeus muscle

Digastric muscle

Hyoid bone

Thyroid cartilage

Cricoid cartilage

Fascia

Foramen magnum

Pharyngeal tubercle

Superior pharyngeal constrictor muscle

Middle pharyngeal constrictor muscle

Inferior pharyngeal constrictor muscle

Posterior view

Figure 4-4. Constrictors of the throat.

The superior pharyngeal constrictor is continuous with buccinator; it arises from the pterygomandibular raphe and the upper and lower jaws and curves upward and backward to insert into the median pharyngeal raphe. The middle pharyngeal constrictor, the smallest constrictor muscle, arises from the hyoid bone and fans out to attach to the median raphe, its upper fibers overlapping those of the superior constrictor. The inferior pharyngeal constrictor arises from the oblique ridge of the thyroid cartilage and curves upward and backward to insert into the median raphe, its upper fibers overlapping those of the middle constrictor. The

lowest part of the inferior constrictor is the cricopharyngeus muscle (Fig. 4-3), which arises from the cricoid cartilage and, as we've seen, functions as one of the extrinsic muscles of the larynx. This muscle anchors the cricoid cartilage directly backward to the esophagus, which begins at this point just behind the cricoid.

The constrictors are responsible for swallowing. Though technically not considered as sphincter muscles, they constrict in turn during swallowing to draw the bolus of food downward until it reaches the esophagus, which conveys the food in peristaltic waves into the stomach.

The Function of the Palate

The palate has two sections: the hard palate in front and the soft palate, or velum, in back (Fig. 4-2). The main function of the hard palate is to separate the nasal passageway from the mouth. This makes it possible for an infant to breathe while suckling, and for an adult to chew food while still breathing through the nose.

The soft palate is a movable fold that functions as a valve that can close off or open the nasal port, the opening between the nasal passage and the pharynx. It hangs behind the hard palate and forms an incomplete septum, or divide, between the mouth and pharynx. It is made up of an underlying flap of aponeurotic or fibrous tissue attaching to the back end of the hard palate, forming a kind of veil at the back of the throat (hence the name velum, which means "veil" in Latin). Muscle fibers join into it from above and below, and it is covered with mucous membrane.

The soft palate can be likened to a diaphragm that is capable of being raised or depressed, and serves a number of functions. When the soft palate is raised, it presses upon the back of the superior constrictor of the throat at a region called "Passavant's cushion," sealing off the nasopharynx, or nasal port (Fig. 4-5a). When the body of the tongue is raised and presses against the soft palate, this closes off the oral cavity from the pharynx, making it possible to breathe exclusively through the nostrils while chewing (Fig. 4-5b). Since we are designed to breathe through our nostrils (which filter, moisten, and warm the air) and to feed through our mouths, this is also the basic "resting position" of the tongue during normal breathing. When the nasal port is closed and the velum and tongue create an oral seal, both the nasal and oral cavities are sealed off from the pharynx; this happens when we hold our breath and swim under water. In this case, neither water nor air can pass through the nasal and oral cavities into the pharynx (Fig. 4-5c). During swallowing, the palate is first raised in order to close the nasal port and allow food to enter the pharynx. It is then depressed against the raised tongue to drive the food downward during the act of swallowing.

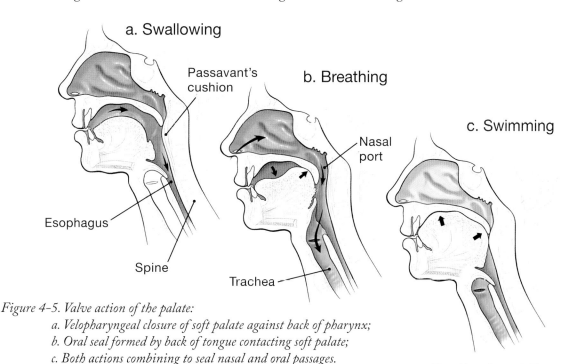

Figure 4-5. Valve action of the palate:
    a. Velopharyngeal closure of soft palate against back of pharynx;
    b. Oral seal formed by back of tongue contacting soft palate;
    c. Both actions combining to seal nasal and oral passages.

The Muscles of the Palate

There are five muscles of the palate. Acting on the palate from above are the muscles that tighten and elevate the palate (Fig. 4-6). Levator veli palatini is a thick muscle that arises from the temporal bones on either side of the skull and, passing obliquely downward and inward, joins into the soft palate at its midline, where it blends with the fibers of the muscle on the opposite side to form a kind of sling that supports the soft palate. Its function is to move the soft palate upward and backward, closing the velopharyngeal valve or nasal port. When we yawn or deepen the voice, which raises the palate, it is this muscle that comes into play—a crucial one for voice users.

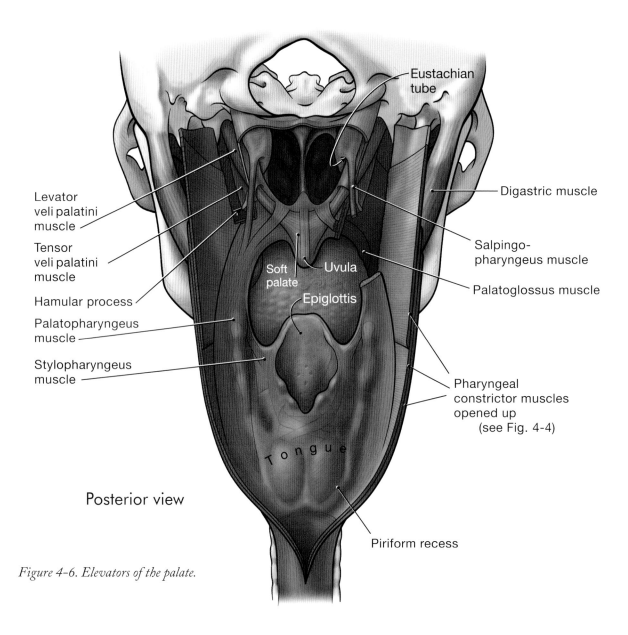

Figure 4–6. Elevators of the palate.

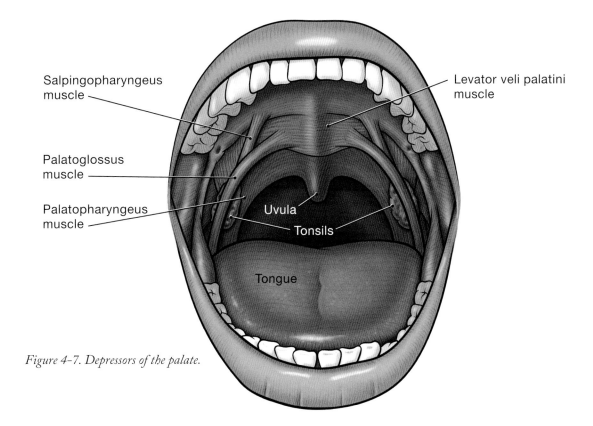

Salpingopharyngeus
muscle

Levator veli palatini
muscle

Palatoglossus
muscle

Palatopharyngeus
muscle

Uvula

Tonsils

Tongue

Figure 4-7. Depressors of the palate.

Tensor veli palatini descends vertically from the sphenoid bone of the skull, runs round a bony protrusion called the hamular process, and inserts laterally into the aponeurosis of the palate (Fig. 4-6). Because it inserts horizontally into the veil of the soft palate, its contraction tenses or stiffens the veil of the palate when the tongue presses up against it in swallowing. It also acts antagonistically to the elevator of the palate by stiffening in opposition to it, helping to create the arches of the palate.

The salpingopharyngeus muscle is a diminutive muscle that originates from the Eustachian tube near the inner ear and, passing downward, joins with the fibers of the palatopharyngeus muscle. This muscle assists in raising the pharynx (Fig. 4-6).

The uvula is the visible structure hanging down from the soft palate just behind the hard palate. It is supported by muscle fibers but has little real function.

There are two depressors of the palate (Figs. 4-6 and 4-7). Just in front of the uvula are the two arches or pillars of the soft palate, which can be easily seen toward the back of the oral cavity. Palatoglossus, which forms the anterior pillar, arises from the soft palate on either side of the uvula and, sloping downward and outward, inserts into the sides of the tongue.

Palatopharyngeus, which forms the posterior pillar, arises from the soft palate behind the palatoglossus muscle and, passing outward and downward, joins with the fibers of the stylopharyngeus muscle to insert into the posterior border of the thyroid cartilage. Palatopharyngeus and palatoglossus depress the palate during eating and swallowing. They also help to elevate the tongue and larynx during swallowing and vocalization.

The Arched Palate

The action of the palate during speaking and singing is variable but, on the whole, singing requires that the palate be arched or raised.

As we have just seen, viewed from the oral cavity, the palate forms arches that run down into the tongue and pharynx; these arches can easily be seen curving down from the uvula, which is situated at the apex of these pillars. When the throat is tight, the tongue tends to be raised and the jaw also tends to be partly closed (Fig. 4-8b). Conversely, when the arches of the palate are raised, the tongue drops and the larynx descends, opening the throat (Fig. 4-8a).

The arching of the palate is due mainly to the action of the tensors and elevators of the palate, which raise the arches. The palate acts in opposition to the tongue, larynx, and hyoid bone. When the palate is depressed, the tongue and larynx are elevated, constricting the throat as in swallowing. When the palate is raised, the tongue, hyoid bone, and larynx are lowered, opening the throat. This happens during the beginning stages of swallowing, and when we inhale or yawn. With a minimal amount of practice, one can learn to raise the arches of the palate at will, bringing them under conscious control.

Arching the palate has a crucial effect on the shape of the vocal tract. Because the palate forms a septum separating the oral cavity from the pharynx, a depressed or collapsed palate separates the oral and pharyngeal cavities. In contrast, arching the palate unifies the oral cavity and pharynx by making them into a continuous resonator and is thus a crucial element in skillfully shaping the vocal tract in singing (see Figs. 4-12a and b).

In singing, the nasal port is mainly kept open, particularly during vowel production and when singing in the upper registers. This means that the palate is actually kept fairly low, not high, as singers often claim.

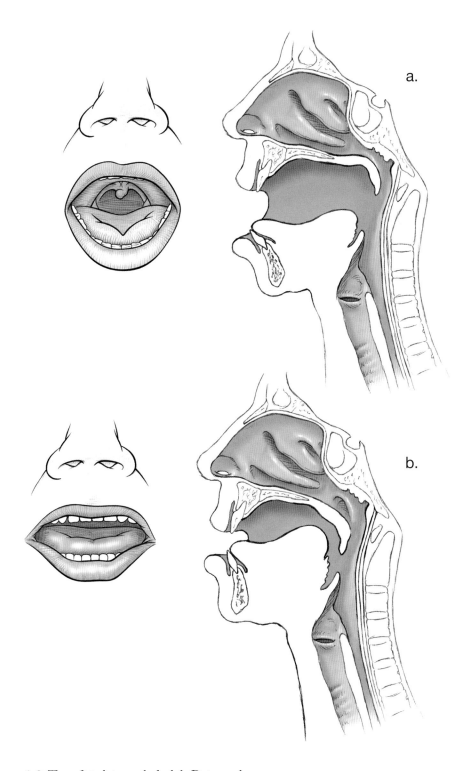

Figure 4-8. The soft palate: a. Arched; b. Depressed.

The Tongue and Its Function

The tongue, or lingual region, is composed of intrinsic muscle fibers that form the body or dorsum of the tongue itself, as well as four extrinsic muscles whose fibers join with the dorsum of the tongue and move it from points outside the dorsum of the tongue (Fig. 4-9). The tongue lies at the floor of the mouth, and the hyoglossus and genioglossus muscles attach it to the hyoid bone. The tongue is divided down its midline by a fibrous septum and is made up of several layers of muscle fibers running in various directions. The superficial layer is the superior longitudinal muscle. The middle layer is composed of vertical and transverse muscles. The deepest layer is the inferior longitudinal muscle. These intrinsic muscles intermingle with the fibers of the extrinsic muscles that join into the dorsum of the tongue—in particular, the styloglossus and hyoglossus muscles on the sides of the tongue and the genioglossus muscle on its underside. This complex arrangement of intrinsic fibers makes it possible to shorten the tongue, to form it into a convex or concave shape (with the tip of the tongue turned upward), to narrow and elongate the tongue, or to flatten and broaden it. In conjunction with the extrinsic muscles that move and position the tongue, this complex arrangement of fibers also makes it possible to form the sounds of speech.

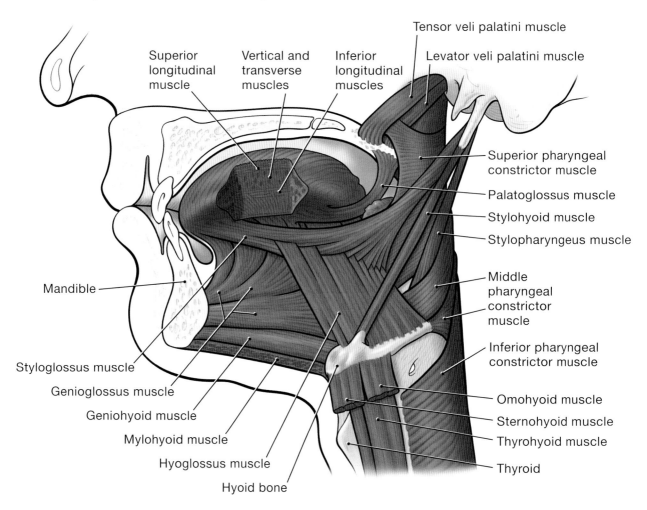

Figure 4-9. The tongue and its muscles.

As we have seen, the extrinsic muscles of the tongue lie below the dorsum and move the tongue in various directions (Fig. 4-9). The first of these extrinsic muscles is the hyoglossus, which originates from the hyoid bone and passes vertically upward and forward to insert into the sides of the tongue. Genioglossus runs vertically from the inner side of the symphysis of the jaw and spreads out in a fan-like shape on either side of the midline of the jaw to insert into the underside of the tongue along its whole length and to the hyoid bone. The styloglossus muscle originates at the styloid process and joins into both sides of the body of the tongue and with the fibers of the hyoglossus muscle. The styloglossus muscle draws the tongue upward and backward. The palatoglossus muscle arises from the soft palate and, passing down and forward, inserts into the sides of the tongue. Its function is to draw the base of the tongue upward and to compress the palate during swallowing. The extrinsic muscles make it possible to move the tongue as a whole, as in sucking or positioning food in the mouth, and play an important role in the action of swallowing.

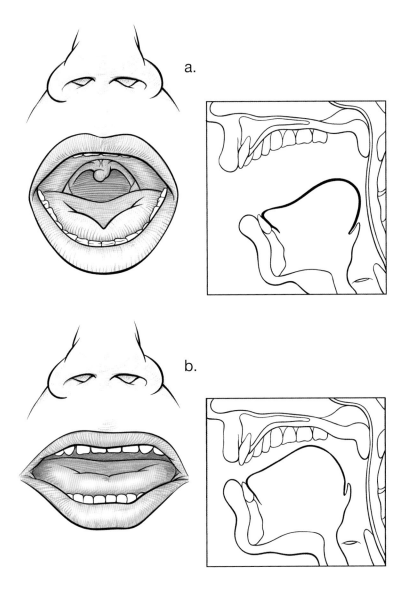

Figure 4-10. a. Position of the tongue during singing: open throat; b. Raised position of tongue: closed throat.

Position of the Tongue in Singing

In singing, the throat functions best when it is open. This means, among other things, that the tongue must remain fairly low in the mouth with the tip touching the lower teeth, the tongue lowest in front, and the jaw open and relaxed. This is easiest to experience when producing the "ah" vowel, which involves the least manipulation of the tongue and is therefore the default vowel in singing. In this relaxed position the tongue also tends naturally to form a groove down the midline (Fig. 4-10).

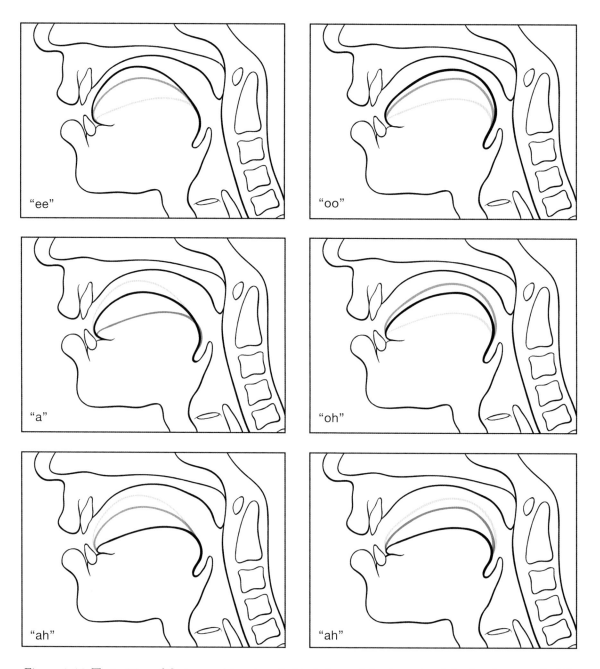

"ee"

"oo"

"a"

"oh"

"ah"

"ah"

Figure 4-11. The position of the tongue determines the kind of vowel that is produced. In the column on the left, the tongue is positioned forward, producing the so-called "front" vowels (ee, a as in "hay," ah); in the column on the right, the tongue is positioned toward the back of the throat, producing the "back" vowels (oo, oh, ah).

The tongue is also the most important factor in the formation of vowels. The default vowel is "ah," because in the absence of trying to form a vowel, "ah" is what you'll get. The other vowels involve a change of position of the tongue. Singers tend to change only the tongue position and not to involve the lips and mouth too much, as these cause unnecessary tension (Fig. 4-11).

Producing the open quality required in singing is also related to vowel sounds. To maintain an open throat, singers often alter spoken vowel sounds, tending to make them open and darker, as when we yawn and open the throat on the vowel sound. In covered singing, the larynx is lowered so that both the aperture to, and the lowest part of, the larynx are widened. So tongue position, vowel formation, and the lowered larynx are all crucial factors in singing.

The Low Larynx and Widened Pharynx

The final element of an open throat is the low position of the larynx. In Chapter Three, we saw that a skilled singer does not appreciably raise the larynx but, by engaging the suspensory muscles of the larynx, is able to maintain the larynx in a low position even while singing in the higher registers. This keeps the larynx free in its operation so that it does not constrict as the pitch rises. It also assists the larynx in producing a supported falsetto tone and head voice.

Maintaining a low larynx has another effect as well: it lengthens the vocal tract and widens the lower part of the pharynx. This tends to produce a more open vowel quality, which sounds darker as a consequence. Sometimes called "covering," this quality is a critical part of classical vocal training and is largely due to the action of the suspensory muscles, which tend to open the throat as the larynx is lowered. One of the muscles responsible for opening the pharynx is the paired stylopharyngeus muscles, which are farther apart at their origins than at their insertions (see Fig. 4-4), and which therefore pull the walls of the pharynx apart as they pull upward, dilating the throat. Their action is opposed by the depressors of the larynx, which maintain the low position of the larynx and thus lengthen the vocal tract as it widens (Fig. 4-12).

Lengthening and widening this part of the vocal tract is one of the most important elements in modulating the voice. The sound that emanates from the vibrating vocal folds is a complex tone composed of a fundamental frequency, or pitch, and a number of overtones, which give the tone a rich and complex timbre. The cavities above the larynx act as a flexible resonator for this vocal signature, augmenting certain frequencies and attenuating others. The vocal tract has several resonance frequencies that maximally augment the vocal signal, and the lowered larynx and widened pharynx in particular produce a formant, not found in the average speaking voice, that matches perfectly with the frequency of the vibrations from the larynx. This creates the powerful, ringing tones of the operatic voice that can carry over an orchestra and in large spaces. Sometimes called the "singer's formant," this quality is prized by classical and operatic singers and achieving it constitutes a large part of their training.

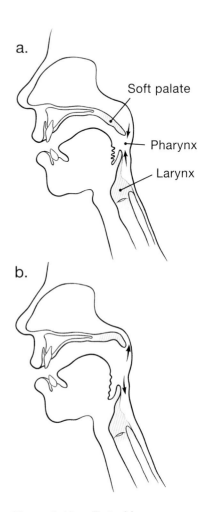

a.

Soft palate

Pharynx

Larynx

b.

Figure 4-12. a. Raised larynx and constricted throat; b. Lowered larynx and open throat. Notice that in (a), the soft palate and larynx move toward each other and the pharynx is shortened; in (b), the soft palate and larynx move away from each other and the pharynx is lengthened.

Although the facial bones and muscles do not play a direct role in phonation, they nevertheless form a crucial component of the vocal instrument. There are several reasons for this. First, the facial muscles are organs of communication and expression. Second, we often "collapse" the vocal mechanism as part of losing tone in the face, sleeping with the mouth open, using the voice in a "heavy" way, collapsing the palate; as a result, many voice users develop throatiness of tone and other vocal problems over time. Toning the facial muscles is an essential component in "activating" the vocal instrument, as many singers, who maintain healthy and youthful tone in the facial muscles well into old age, know well. Third, vocal function is directly influenced by tone of the facial muscles, which have indirect reflex connections with the larynx and throat; learning to "place" the voice by toning the facial muscles can profoundly influence both the larynx and the throat.

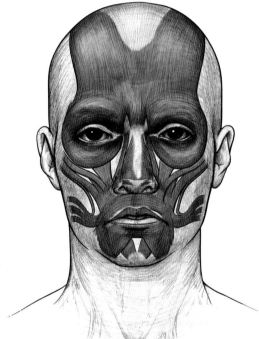

Figure 5-1. Muscles of the face.

The facial muscles are different from other skeletal muscles because they do not attach from one bone to another but, in most cases, arise from bone or cartilage and insert into the integument, or skin tissue, often blending with the fibers of other muscles. This gives them the ability to produce facial expressions by moving the skin, to narrow or wrinkle areas of skin and tissue, and to move or contract apertures, as in the case of the area around the eyes. In particular, the areas around the mouth, the lateral region of the orbits of the eyes, and the region between the eyes are convergence points for muscles whose fibers tend to blend with one another. Because the facial muscles are often overlapping and are continuous with the fascia covering the face and neck, they form a movable sheet of connective tissue covering the entire face (Fig. 5-1).

The Mask

Perhaps because singers experience vibrations in the nasal region, this region of the face—often referred to as the singer's "mask"—has often been considered one of the key vocal resonators. Although neither the nasal bones nor the nasal cavities actually participate in the resonance of the voice, the practice of "placing" the voice in the mask does affect the function of the larynx and produce more focus and ring in the voice. The "mask" is made up mainly of the maxilla, the nasal bones, and the lower part of the frontal bone where the sinuses are located; singers are usually aware of this region while singing (Fig. 5-2).

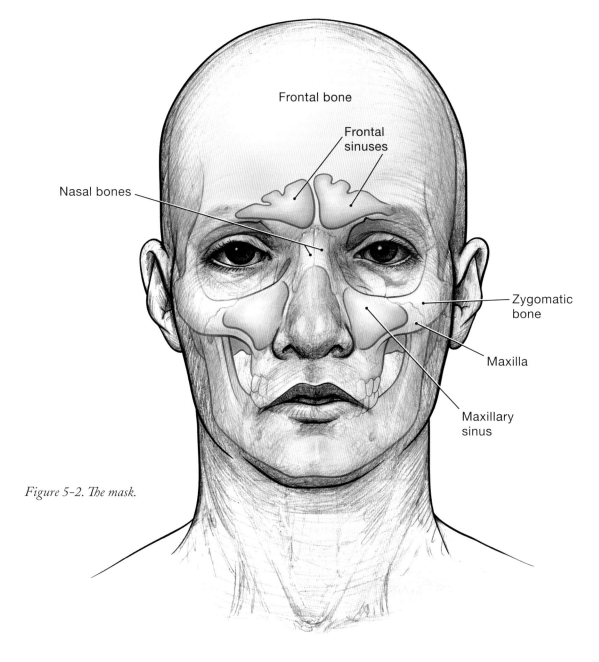

Figure 5-2. The mask.

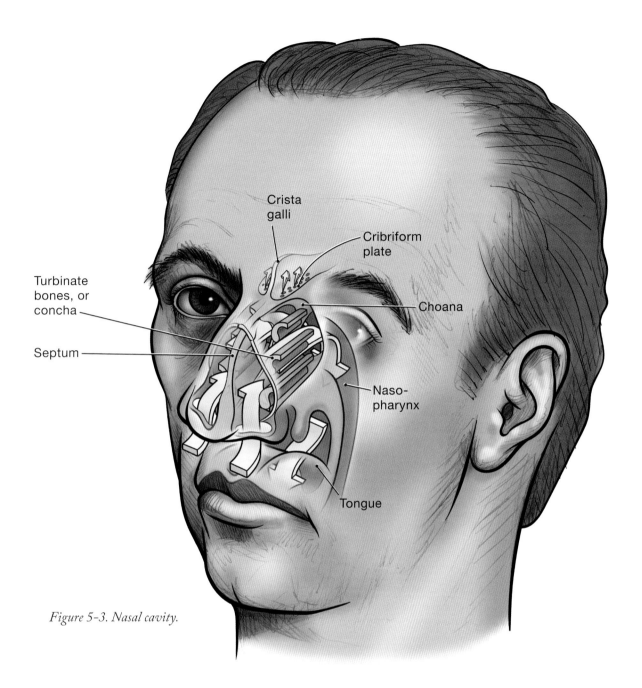

Figure 5-3. Nasal cavity.

Labels on figure:
- Crista galli
- Cribriform plate
- Choana
- Turbinate bones, or concha
- Septum
- Naso-pharynx
- Tongue

The Nostrils and Nasal Cavity

The nostrils are the primary breathing channel during normal breathing. The nostrils open into the nasal cavities or fossae, which are formed by the winged turbinate bones of the skull (also called conchae) separated by a septum into two separate cavities (Fig. 5-3). These cavities, in addition to being lined with mucous membranes with a rich vascular supply, separate into olfactory and respiratory sections. Two apertures (or choanae) at the posterior part of these cavities open into the nasopharynx. In addition to functioning as a sensory organ for smell, the nostrils moisten, filter, and warm the air taken into the lungs.

Muscles of the Nostrils

Dilating and activating the nostrils is associated with inhalation, which in turn tends to open the throat. There are three dilators and three depressors of the nostrils (Fig. 5-4). Levator labii superioris alaeque nasi (from Latin, meaning "elevator of the upper lip next to the nose") originates from the upper portion of the maxilla near the inner margin of the orbit of the eye. Angling downward and outward, some of its fibers attach to the upper lip and some to the cartilage of the ala nasi (the wing-like portion of the nostril, from the Latin ala, meaning "wing"). It elevates the upper lip, and elevates and dilates the ala, as in producing a sneer.

Just beneath levator labii superioris alaeque nasi is dilatator naris posterior. It arises from the margin of the nasal notch of the maxilla (see Fig. 5-7) and inserts into the skin near the margin of the ala. Dilatator naris anterior arises from the cartilage of the ala and attaches to the skin near its margin. These muscles, as their names suggest, dilate the alae.

The nasalis muscle, which has a transverse and alar part, is the compressor of the nostrils. The transverse part, also known as compressor nasi or naris, originates at the maxilla next to the ala; its fibers expand upward and inward just behind the nostrils and blend into the fascia of the cartilage of the nose, which is continuous with that of the procerus muscle on the bridge of the nose. The alar part of the nasalis muscle (in Gray's, the outer part of the depressor alae nasi) arises from the maxilla below the origin of the transverse part of the nasalis muscle and inserts into the septum and posterior part of the ala. The function of these two muscles is to draw the alae downward and to constrict them.

The depressor septi nasi muscle (in Gray's, the inner part of depressor alae nasi) arises from the maxilla under the nose and inserts into the septum and posterior part of the ala. Its function is to draw the alae downward and to constrict them.

Compressor narium minor is a tiny muscle arising from the cartilage of the ala and attaching to the skin at the tip of the nose. It also depresses the cartilage of the nose and compresses the nostrils.

The action of these muscles is related to the soft palate and opening the throat in singing. Compressing the nostrils tends to be associated with depressing and collapsing the palate; dilating the nostrils and sneering, which are associated with inspiration, tend to raise the palate and dilate the pharynx. Think of sneering and smelling something pungent, and notice how this enlivens and dilates the nostrils and even helps to open the throat.

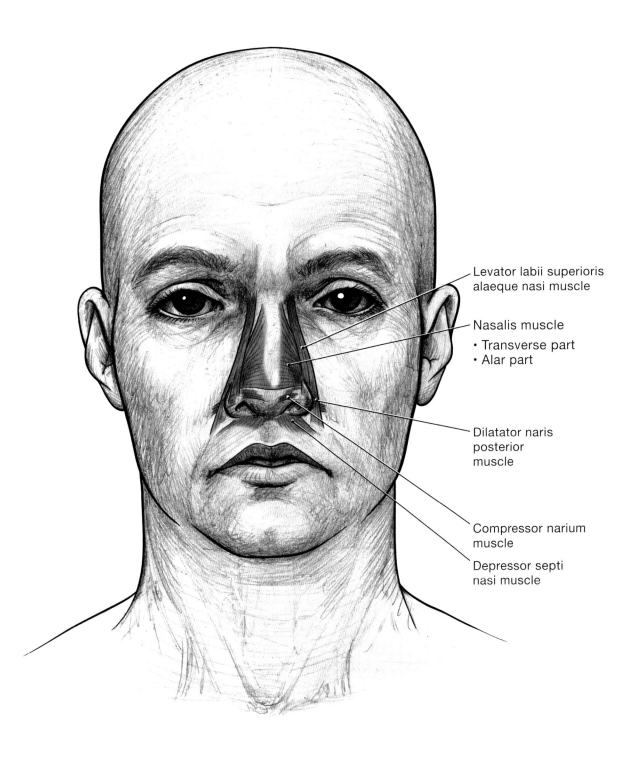

Levator labii superioris
alaeque nasi muscle

Nasalis muscle
• Transverse part
• Alar part

Dilatator naris
posterior
muscle

Compressor narium
muscle

Depressor septi
nasi muscle

Figure 5-4. Muscles of the nose.

The Eyes and Forehead

Although the eyes are organs of perception, they are also expressive of mood and communicate feelings, and are in this sense crucial to the vocal organ. There are several muscles of the eyes and forehead (Fig. 5-5). The key forehead muscle, frontalis, draws the scalp back, raising the eyebrows and wrinkling the forehead. It is actually part of a tendinous sheet that runs right over the scalp to the occiput in back, where there is another section of muscle tissue (not pictured).

Corrugator supercilii lies in between the eyebrows; it is the frowning muscle and causes the vertical wrinkles in the forehead. It arises from the inner part of the brow, or superciliary ridge of the frontal bone, running outward to insert into the skin above the orbit.

Procerus (also called pyramidalis nasi) lies between the eyebrows. It arises from the cartilage on the upper part of the nose and the fascia over the nasal bone and inserts into the skin and the muscle fibers of the frontalis muscle. This muscle draws the eyebrows together and also produces frowning. The fibers of the frontalis muscle are continuous with corrugator supercilii, procerus, and orbicularis oculi.

Surrounding the orbits of the eyes and eyelids is a sphincter muscle, orbicularis oculi. Its outer ring of fibers is the orbital part; the inner ring, covering the outer eyelid, is the palpebral part. Orbicularis oculi arises from the frontal and nasal part of the maxilla bone, its fibers fanning out above and below to cover the eyelids and to encircle the orbits of the eyes to the cheek and temples. Its function is to narrow and protect the area around the eyes and, along with the frowning muscles, to produce squinting. The palpebral portion closes the eyelids. Continual contraction of the orbital region tends to produce permanent squinting of the eyes, drawing the eyebrow over the eyelid.

Because we communicate with the face and eyes, habitual frowning, worry, and seriousness of demeanor cause the eyes to lose tone and expressiveness, which in turn signifies loss of energy or collapse of the vocal organ. The orbicularis oculi muscles become habitually tightened from squinting and tension. We also tend to become "glazed over" and hypnotic when concentrating on our work or sitting at a computer, which hardens the eyes and lowers muscle tone around the eyes. Softening and brightening the eyes tends to relax and tone the area around the eyes and is associated with a more positive mental attitude and activated vocal instrument. Although associated with smiling, the best way to bring this about is not to force a smile but by thinking of something humorous or touching, by making eye contact with another person, or by looking attentively at an object.

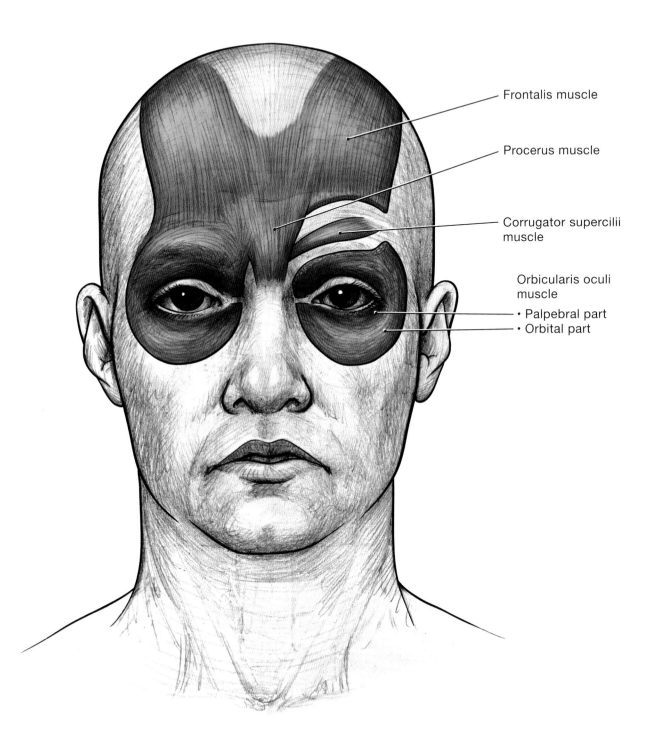

Frontalis muscle

Procerus muscle

Corrugator supercilii
muscle

Orbicularis oculi
muscle
• Palpebral part
• Orbital part

Figure 5-5. Muscles of the eyes and forehead.

The Cheeks

The cheek muscles are also associated with activation of the vocal instrument and with a more focused tone. There are several muscles around the cheek and the area above the upper lip that relate to facial expressions such as sadness and laughing (Fig. 5-6). Levator labii superioris arises from the lower margin of the orbit formed by the zygomatic and maxilla bones. It passes downward and inward to converge into the muscular fibers around the mouth. Its function is to elevate the upper lip.

Levator anguli oris arises from the ridge of the canine tooth on the maxilla bone, just where the cheekbone, or zygomatic bone, begins to protrude. It passes downward to blend into the muscular fibers of orbicularis oris and zygomaticus major, around the mouth. Its function is to raise the angle of the lips. You can feel the effects of these muscles if you crinkle the nose, which engages the elevators to bunch up the cheeks just below the eyes.

Zygomaticus minor arises from the zygomatic, or cheekbone, and passes downward and inward to converge, with levator labii superioris, into the muscular fibers of orbicularis oris. It draws the mouth upward and slightly back, as in expressing sadness.

Zygomaticus major arises from the arch of the cheekbone where it curves to form the lateral plane of the face. It passes obliquely downward and forward to insert into orbicularis oris next to levator anguli oris. It draws the corners of the mouth back, as in laughing. Where zygomaticus major originates in front of the ear, it tends to be continuous along the lateral plane of the face with the muscle in front of the ear, auricularis anterior muscle, as well as the temporomandibular joint.

Because of the tendency to lose expressiveness in the face, it is useful to tone the cheek muscles by "brightening" the eyes and raising or rounding the cheeks. Toning the eyes and cheek muscles helps to activate the suspensory muscles of the larynx and to "place" the voice forward, giving it a brighter tone. This also helps to maintain healthy muscle tone and youthfulness in the facial muscles well into old age. When muscular tension in the eyes and cheeks is reduced, you can feel the musculature of the face become mobile and free right around to the sides of the face and jaw, which helps to open and tone the muscles of the palate and throat.

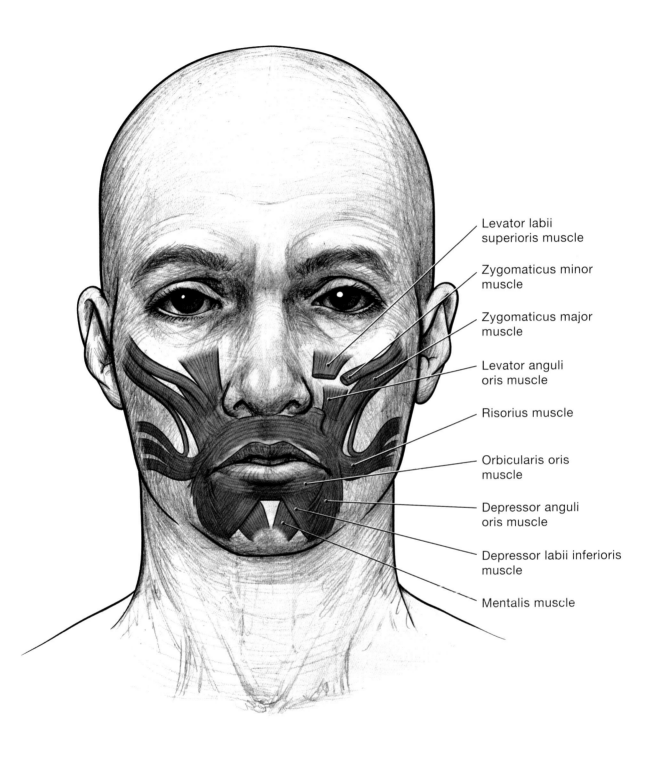

Levator labii
superioris muscle

Zygomaticus minor
muscle

Zygomaticus major
muscle

Levator anguli
oris muscle

Risorius muscle

Orbicularis oris
muscle

Depressor anguli
oris muscle

Depressor labii inferioris
muscle

Mentalis muscle

Figure 5-6. Muscles of the cheek and mouth.

The Jaw and Temporomandibular Joint

The jaw or mandible (also called the inferior maxillary bone) is the largest bone of the face (Fig. 5-7). The section of the jaw that forms the chin is called the symphysis; the main line of the jaw is the body; the upward extension that forms the joint and attachments for muscles is the ramus. The ramus divides into the coronoid process in front and the condylar process in back. The coronoid process serves as the point of attachment for the temporalis muscle; the condylar process articulates with the temporal bone to form the temporomandibular joint.

The temporomandibular joint is located directly in front of the external acoustic meatus, the opening for the ear (Fig. 5-7). Directly in front of this opening is a depression called the mandibular fossa. The condyles of the jaw sit within this depression and, when they rotate, produce the basic hinging action of the jaw. The condyles can also glide forward in relation to the mandibular fossa so that the jaw as a whole can move forward and back. When one condyle moves forward and the other moves backward, the jaw produces a grinding motion.

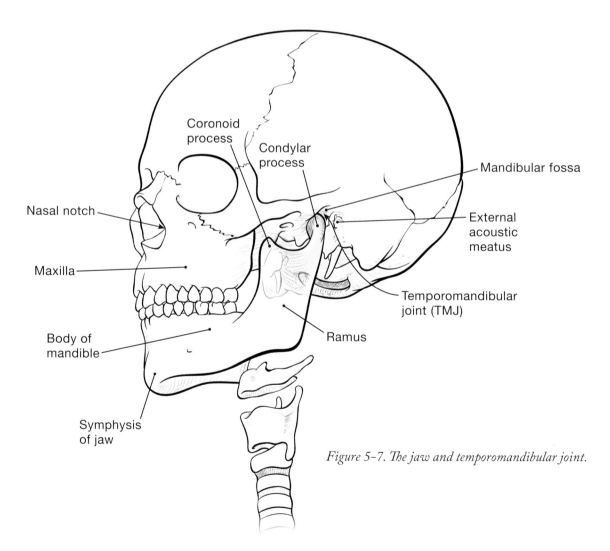

Figure 5-7. The jaw and temporomandibular joint.

The temporomandibular joint is basically a gliding hinge joint. Between the mandibular fossa and the condyle is a cartilage called the articular disc. On its lower surface the articular disc forms a rounded surface that cradles the condyle, which is able to rotate within this disc, producing the hinging action of the jaw (Fig. 5-8a). This disc, however, is not fixed to the temporal bone but is lubricated on its upper surface with synovial fluid so that it can glide forward in relation to the mandibular fossa, bringing the condyle and jaw with it (Fig. 5-8b).

The temporomandibular joint, then, is really two joints: the hinge joint formed by the articulation of the condyle with the articular disc, and the gliding joint formed by the articulation of the articular disc with the temporal bone. Both articulations are lubricated, and the entire joint is enclosed within a capsular ligament and supported by two other ligaments. The jaw is also supported by the stylomandibular ligament (not pictured), which extends from the styloid process of the temporal bone to the angle of the jaw.

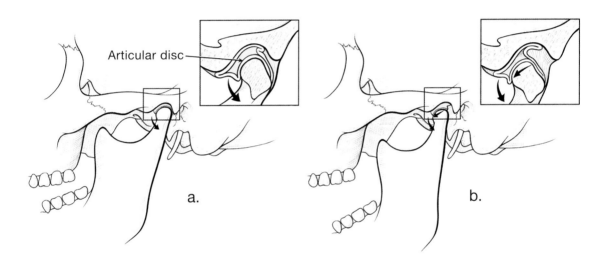

Figure 5-8. a. Partial opening of the jaw for speaking: the jaw hinges at the joint (downward arrow) without moving forward in space; b. Wider opening of the jaw for singing: the jaw swings or moves forward in relation to the temporal bone (forward arrow) as it hinges to open (downward arrow).

Position of the Jaw in Singing

Normal speech does not require that the jaw be opened widely; the condyles of the jaw rotate within the articular disc but no other movement takes place. For the purposes of singing, however, the jaw should open more fully so that the sound is not blocked and to create a large enough oral cavity for efficient resonance. In this case the jaw must not only hinge at the condyle but must also glide forward; otherwise the condyle gets jammed and the jaw cannot open freely (Fig. 5-8b). When the condyle glides forward, you can feel a pocket open in front of the lower ear. Allowing the jaw to open freely is unfamiliar to many voice users, who habitually tighten and retract the jaw.

Muscles of the Jaw

Three muscles produce the grinding, chewing, and snapping actions of the jaw (Fig. 5-9). Temporalis, which is a broad, powerful muscle that originates broadly at the temporal region on the side of the head and converges to insert into the coronoid process of the jaw, is mainly responsible for the snapping action of the jaw. The masseter muscle originates at the cheekbone and inserts into the ramus of the jaw. Its function is to raise the lower jaw and to clamp it shut.

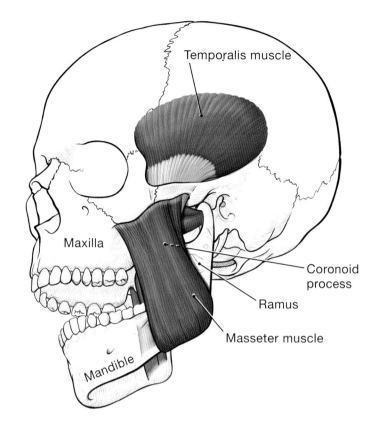

Figure 5-9. Muscles of the jaw.

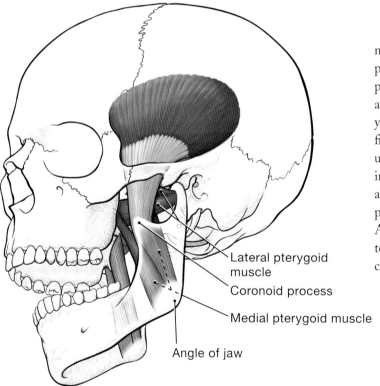

The lateral and medial pterygoid muscles arise from the cheekbone and palate areas of the skull. The medial pterygoid inserts into the ramus and angle of the jaw bone. The lateral pterygoid inserts into the interarticular fibrocartilage of the temporomandibular joint, and is the principal agent in drawing the jaw forward. When acting alternately, the function of the pterygoid muscles is to grind the jaw. All three of the jaw muscles acting together produce the movements of chewing and grinding food.

Three muscles depress or open the jaw, all of them on the underside of the jaw (Fig. 5-10). Digastricus, which means "having two bellies," originates at the mastoid process, runs through a loop on the hyoid bone, and continues on to insert into the jaw. Mylohyoid and genio-hyoid form the floor of the jaw and also relate the jaw to the hyoid bone. These two muscles form the floor of the jaw and are sometimes referred to as the "diaphragm of the jaw" (Fig. 5-11). Singers often focus on the large closers of the jaw when seeking to release the jaw. But these jaw muscles evolved as part of the throat muscula-ture attaching to the hyoid bone and sympathetically tighten in response to tension in the throat, which is why the throat muscles are the real key to releasing the muscles of the jaw.

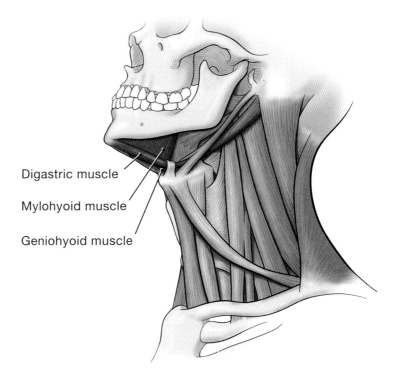

Figure 5-10. Depressors of the jaw.

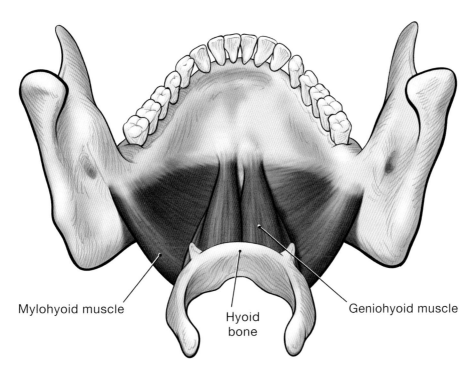

Figure 5-11. The diaphragm of the jaw.

A nyone who has made even a cursory study of the human larynx is likely to assume, based on how beautifully suited it is for producing sound, that most of its remarkable and intricate features evolved mainly for this purpose. In fact, most of the features of the larynx evolved for reasons other than vocal communication. To better understand the design of the larynx and voice in general, let's look in this final chapter at some of the stages by which the larynx and voice evolved.

The Origin of the Larynx

The original function of the larynx was to protect the airway in fish that could breathe air. As we all know, fish do not normally breathe air but take their oxygen out of the water flowing through their gills. Certain species of fish, however, developed lung sacs so that they could gulp in air when they came to the surface, or survive in the mud during dry periods. These lung sacs were accessed by a short passageway that opened from the floor of the pharynx. In order to keep water or food from entering this air passage, the opening was protected by a simple valve, or circular sphincter muscle, that remained closed when the fish was under water or feeding (Fig. 6-1). The human larynx, although greatly modified from this original form, still functions as a sphincter to close off and protect the airway.

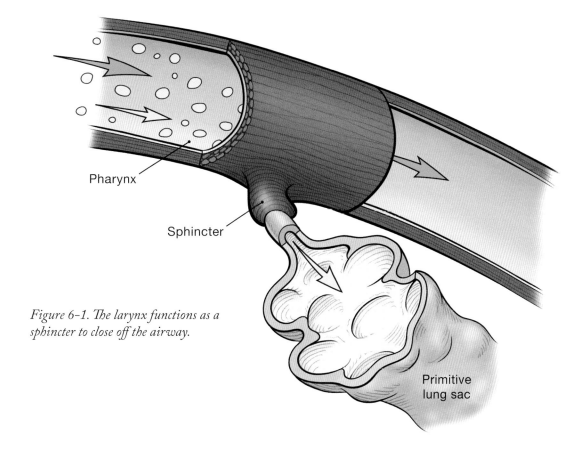

Pharynx

Sphincter

Primitive
lung sac

Figure 6–1. The larynx functions as a sphincter to close off the airway.

Evolution of the Cartilages and Muscles of the Larynx

In fish that have lungs, there is no way of actively opening the sphincter of the larynx; during periods when air was needed, the sphincter simply relaxed and air flowed into the lungs. Animals on land, however, needed to more actively control the opening and closing of the glottis. This was an absolute necessity in animals that breathed by suction, since the sucking action of the rib cage pulled the lips of the glottis, or the opening of the larynx, together and therefore had to be counteracted with muscles and scaffolding that could actively hold it open.

In mammals that developed a sophisticated larynx, these changes happened in several stages. First, muscle fibers attaching close to the sphincter shifted direction in such a way that they could actively pull on the margins of the glottis and dilate or open it. (These were the precursors of the posterior cricoarytenoid muscles.) Next, cartilages appeared along the margins of the glottis; these served as anchors for the dilator muscles, making the pull of the muscles more efficient (Fig. 6-2).

Part of the lateral cartilages formed into the arytenoid cartilages at the posterior of the glottis and served as attachments for the vocal folds; other parts of the cartilage on either side fused to form the cricoid ring at the top of the trachea. The arytenoid cartilages formed joints with the cricoid cartilage; when the arytenoid cartilages swiveled, the rim of the glottis could be actively spread apart.

The thyroid cartilage also appeared in evolution as an outgrowth of the cricoid cartilage. At first the two cartilages were fused, but in higher mammals they separated to form a hinge. Because the thyroarytenoid muscle now attached at its front end to the thyroid cartilage (instead of the cricoid), the movement of the thyroid in relation to the cricoid cartilage shortened the glottis and facilitated its closure.

With the appearance of arytenoid cartilages and muscles that moved it, the glottis was now closed by three sets of muscles and opened by one. The thyroarytenoid muscles formed the lips of the glottis and, by contracting, closed off the glottis directly. Two other muscles, the lateral cricoarytenoids on the side of the cricoid and the transverse arytenoids in back, pulled parts of the arytenoids together to close the glottis. Although modified from its original form, these three muscles still formed a sphincter that closed the glottis; the posterior cricoarytenoid formed the dilator (Fig. 6-3).

The larynx now had many of the basic features we see in humans. The arytenoid, thyroid, and cricoid cartilages served as a framework for muscles that efficiently opened and closed the glottis. The posterior cricoarytenoid muscle abducted the vocal folds. The thyroarytenoid muscles, or vocal folds, were the tensors of the glottis; the lateral cricoarytenoids and the transverse arytenoids were the closers; and the cricothyroid muscles were the stretchers. Being able to both open and close, the larynx now performed the two vital functions of protecting the airway and ensuring a constant supply of air, but it was also well suited as a sound-producing organ.

Extrinsic Muscles of the Larynx and Deglutition

One of the crucial roles of the extrinsic muscles of the larynx is during deglutition, or swallowing. In most reptiles, the larynx lies on the floor of the pharynx and does not obstruct the passage of food, which is bolted in large pieces. In land animals, the larynx tilted up in back so that the airway was in a direct line with the mouth, which placed the trachea and esophagus parallel to each other. This made it easier to get a constant supply of air, but it also increased the danger of aspirating food, since the open airway now lay more directly in the path of the bolus of food. To protect the airway during swallowing, the larynx now not only closed; it was also raised by the suprahyoid muscles, which pulled it up under the tongue. In snakes, the larynx is pulled right up to the teeth, so that the airway remains completely open even while its huge prey is slowly worked down its throat.

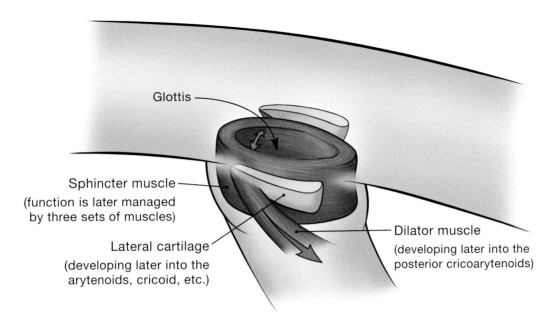

Figure 6-2. Sphincter muscles and dilator.

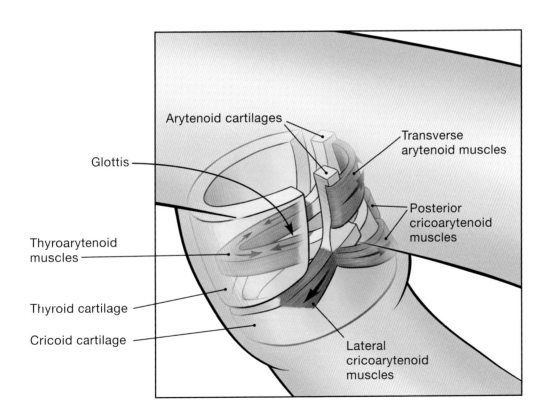

Figure 6-3. Further development of the muscles that dilate and close the airway.

The Palate, Epiglottis, and Nasal Passages

In all animals that breathe, the nasal passage communicates with the air tract so that the flow of air in and out of the lungs can bring molecules into the olfactory organ. In reptiles, air breathed through the nostrils comes directly into the pharynx (Fig. 6-4a). In mammals, a secondary palate formed between the nasal and oral passages in order to separate the food and respiratory passageways, making it possible to bite or chew while continuing to breathe (Fig. 6-4b). This separation became especially important for herbivorous mammals and suckling infants, which feed for long periods and must be able to continue to breathe while doing so. To make it possible to swallow while breathing, herbivores developed a large flap, or epiglottis, at the front of the larynx. The epiglottis forms a collar with high walls along the sides of the larynx, making it possible for liquids (or vegetables in liquid form) to pass around the sides of the larynx and into the esophagus without any danger of aspirating fluids into the airway (Fig. 6-5).

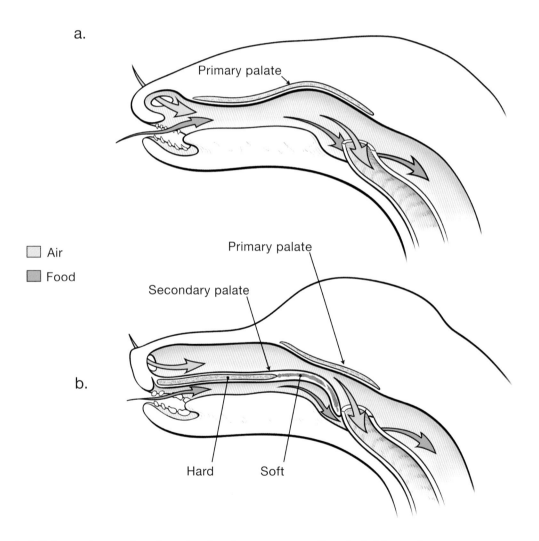

Figure 6-4. Palate and separation of nasal and oral passageways: a. Reptile; b. Mammal.

The epiglottis is also able to make direct contact with the palate, blocking the passage of air through the mouth and directing it through the nose so that the sense of smell can be constantly maintained, even while feeding. (Contrary to popular belief, the epiglottis is not primarily designed to prevent food from entering the larynx; that is the job of the larynx.) In humans, the epiglottis no longer connects with the palate and so has lost its original function. But we are still designed to breathe mainly through the nostrils.

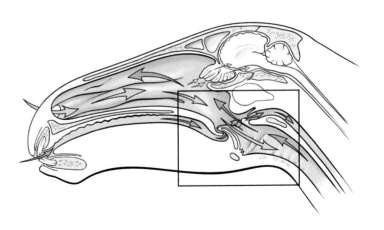

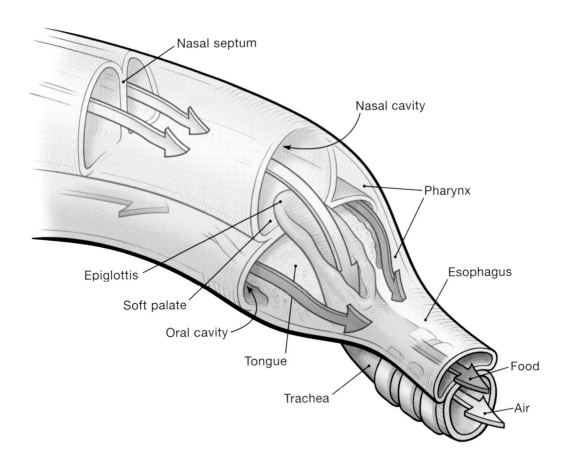

Figure 6-5. Epiglottis and palate in herbivore showing how epiglottis links with palate to close off mouth to breathing.

Design of the Vocal Folds

Another major development in the evolution of the larynx as a sound-producing organ came with the separation of the thyroarytenoid muscles into upper and lower folds. Four-footed animals require a ready supply of air for running but do not need to exert their forelimbs in a strenuous way. Arboreal animals, however, must hang and swing by their powerful forelimbs. Using the arms in this way exerts a tremendous pull on the ribs, which must be stabilized in order for the arm muscles to support the body through the torso. To facilitate this, the thyroarytenoid muscles become separated into upper and lower sections.

The upper folds became downturned and therefore acted as an exit valve that prevented the escape of air when the lungs were filled (Fig. 6-6a). This made it possible, when filling the lungs with air and then trying to exhale by contracting the ribs and abdominal muscles, to raise intrathoracic pressure. (This is useful also during defecation and childbirth, and makes it possible to cough by building up pressure and then suddenly releasing the air.)

The lower folds turned upward, acting as an intake valve that prevented air from coming into the lungs (Fig. 6-6b). This made it possible, by expelling air from the lungs and contracting these lower folds, to create a vacuum that prevented the ribs from rising even when they were pulled upon, creating fixed points for the arm muscles to act upon. The vocal folds now functioned as dual valves for preventing air from coming into and flowing out of the lungs, acting as a regulator of intrathoracic pressure.

The evolution of these dual folds in the thyroarytenoid muscle was a major development in the larynx as a sound-producing organ. The upper folds—called the ventricular bands or false vocal cords because they do not contribute to the production of sound—now functioned nicely as an exit valve for raising intrathoracic pressure. In contrast, the lower folds—called the vocal folds because they vibrate to produce sound—prevented the entrance of air into the lungs but did not oppose the outflow of air, which made them eminently well suited to vibrate freely and to be more finely controlled to produce a greater range of pitches, volume, and different thicknesses, or registers (Fig. 6-6c). In monkeys and other primates, these folds had rather sharp edges, giving the voice a strident tone; when hominids began to walk upright, the vocal folds acquired more rounded edges and became even better suited to the production of sound.

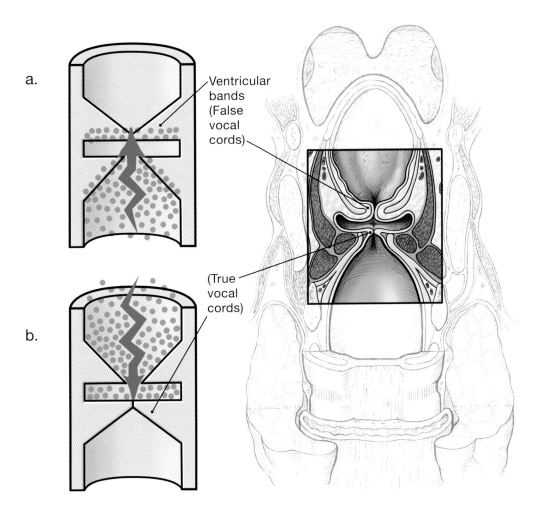

a.

Ventricular bands (False vocal cords)

b.

(True vocal cords)

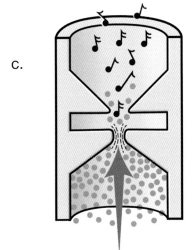

c.

Figure 6-6. a & b. Coronal view of larynx showing inlet and outlet valves (ventricular bands and vocal folds); c. The vocal folds do not oppose the outflow of air and vibrate to produce sound.

The Pharynx, Upright Posture, and Human Speech

Two final developments that must be mentioned in the development of the voice are the evolution of the articulators and the human pharynx. We've already seen that animals that chew food must have a separate passageway for food and breathing. They must also have cheeks for holding the food between the teeth, as well as very movable tongues and lips. Being able to make these movements within a large oral and pharyngeal cavity makes it possible to form a range of vowels as well as to produce the broken-up sounds of human speech, since the tongue, palate, lips, and even the larynx itself are more free for articulation. When animals became arboreal, vision started to take over from olfaction as the primary means of identifying predators; because air no longer needed to be directed through the nose, the epiglottis became decoupled from the palate. This freed these organs for even more efficient phonation and articulation.

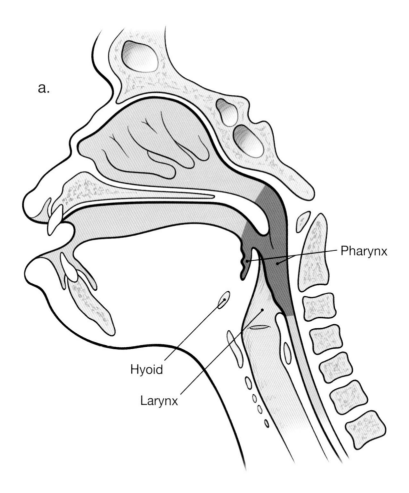

a.

Pharynx

Hyoid

Larynx

Figure 6-7. Pharynx as resonator in: a. Apes; b. Man.

The development of an elongated pharynx is another essential design feature in the vocal system. Most mammals can alter the shape of the oral cavity and lips (as in animals that bark or yelp) but not that of the pharynx. Even in apes, the hyoid bone and larynx lie close to the mouth, so that the pharynx is too short for efficiently producing speech or sustained sounds (Fig. 6-7a). In humans, however, the snout disappears and is replaced with the nose, and the tongue lies farther down the gullet. Since the hyoid bone and larynx are at the base of the tongue, they also move to a lower position, giving humans a longer pharynx than that of apes. Assuming a fully upright posture opened the way for the hyoid bone and larynx to drop still farther, creating an even longer pharynx. This descent of the larynx in humans creates a fully functional pharynx for resonance, speech, and sustained sound (Fig. 6-7b). We still raise the larynx to protect the airway during swallowing, but its lower position is a crucial component of the singing and speaking voice.

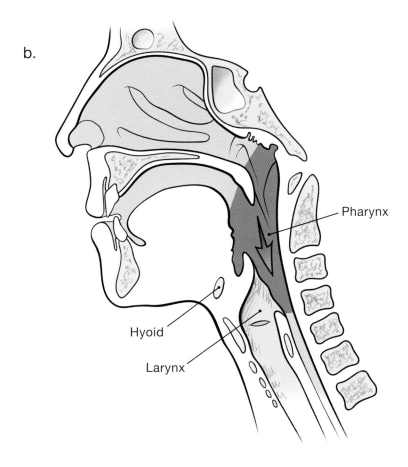

EPILOGUE

The human voice is one of nature's greatest marvels. As we've seen, the vocal instrument is made up of multiple systems, including the respiratory system, the larynx, the throat, the vocal tract, and the face and jaw.

Although the larynx is the primary sound-producing organ, we would not be able to make sound without the flow of air from the lungs, which provides the power source that sets the vocal cords into motion.

The second component of the voice is the larynx, which includes the housing for the vocal cords and the vocal cords themselves. It is here that we are able to bring the vocal folds together and apart, to stretch them, and to tense or tighten them. These actions are produced by the intrinsic muscles of the larynx, which are rather complex but begin to make sense when we look at what actions are performed and how the different muscles produce them.

The larynx itself is suspended within a network of muscles—sometimes called the extrinsic muscles of the larynx—that move the larynx when we swallow and also help it to close up. When we vocalize, these muscles act upon the larynx to assist the vocal folds in stretching, and also aid in the shaping of the vocal tract.

The fourth basic system is the vocal tract, which forms a resonator that augments the sound coming from the vibrating vocal cords. Because the vocal tract is not fixed in shape but can be altered by how we use the different structures such as the mouth, tongue, larynx, and palate, understanding its anatomy is crucial for voice users.

The final system is the face and jaw, which play a crucial role in placing the voice and influence the functioning of the throat and larynx.

Our breathing, the valve of the larynx, the suspensory musculature of the throat, the vocal tract, the lips, face, and tongue—all these structures form a remarkable system whose sensitivity and control are hard to fathom. Working together, these systems cooperate to produce one of nature's greatest marvels, the human voice.

INDEX

A

Abdominal muscles, 14–15
Adam's apple, 27
Alveoli, 22
Aorta, 10
Aryepiglottic folds, 28
Aryepiglottic muscle, 31, 32
Arytenoid cartilages, 26, 27, 29

B

Breathing. *See also* Lungs
    auxiliary muscles of, 16
    definition of, 1
    diaphragm as main muscle of, 10, 12–13
    epiglottis and, 90–91
    functions of, 1
    rib movement and, 1–2, 6–9, 17
    tongue during, 63
Buccinator, 61

C

Cartilages of Santorini. *See* Corniculate cartilages
Cartilages of Wrisberg. *See* Cuneiform cartilages
Cheeks, muscles of, 80–81
Chest register, 43
Compressor narium minor muscle, 76, 77
Conus elasticus, 30, 31
Corniculate cartilages, 27, 28
Coronoid process, 82
Corrugator supercilii muscle, 78, 79
Costal arch, 3
Costovertebral joints, 4, 5
Covering, 71
Cricoarytenoid joint, 28
Cricoid cartilage, 26, 27, 28, 29, 31
Cricopharyngeus muscle, 48, 49, 50, 53, 61, 62
Cricothyroid membrane, 26, 30
Cricothyroid muscle, 34, 40, 42, 50, 51, 52, 53
Cuneiform cartilages, 26, 27, 28

D

Deglutition. *See* Swallowing
Depressor anguli oris muscle, 81
Depressor labii inferioris muscle, 81
Depressor septi nasi muscle, 76, 77
Diaphragm
    abdominal cavity and, 13
    action of, 12
    anatomy of, 10–11
    breathing and, 10
    etymology of, 4, 10
    movement of, 2
    as partition, 4
Digastric muscle, 56, 57, 85
Dilatator naris posterior muscle, 76, 77

E

Epiglottis, 26, 27, 28, 30, 32–33, 90–91
Esophagus, 22, 23
External abdominal oblique muscle, 14, 15
Eyes, muscles of, 78–79

F

Face, muscles of, 73
False cords. *See* Ventricular bands
Falsctto
    action of larynx muscles in, 44
    supported, 53
Forehead, muscles of, 78–79
Frontalis muscle, 78, 79

G

Genioglossus muscle, 68, 69
Geniohyoid muscle, 50, 51, 54, 56, 57, 85
Glottis, 35, 38, 39, 42

H

Head voice, 45, 53
Heart, 4, 10, 11
Hyoglossus muscle, 50, 51, 57, 68, 69
Hyoid bone
    anatomy of, 54
    functions of, 55
    location of, 54
    muscles of, 56–58

I

Inferior pharyngeal constrictor muscle, 61, 62
Inferior thyroarytenoids, 30
Intercostal muscles, 7–9, 14, 17, 18
Internal abdominal oblique muscle, 15

J

Jaw
    diaphragm of, 85
    muscles of, 56–58, 84–85
    position of, in singing, 83
    sections of, 82
    temporomandibular joint and, 82–83
Joint capsule, 26

L

Laryngeal pouch, 31
Laryngopharynx, 60
Larynx
    evolution of, 88, 95
    extrinsic muscles of, 47–48, 88
    false elevators of, 57
    framework of, 26–28
    functions of, 25
    interior of, 30–31
    intrinsic muscles of, 34–45
    joints of, 28–29
    low, 71

    origin of, 87
    structure of, 25, 26
Lateral cricoarytenoid muscle, 36, 38
Lateral pterygoid muscle, 84
Latissimus dorsi muscle, 21
Levator anguli oris muscle, 80, 81
Levator costae muscle, 8
Levatores costarum brevis muscle, 8
Levatores costarum longus muscle, 8
Levator labii superioris alaeque nasi muscle, 76, 77
Levator labii superioris muscle, 80, 81
Levator scapulae muscle, 20
Levator veli palatini muscle, 66, 67
Linea alba, 14, 15
Lungs
    anatomy of, 22
    capacity of, 24
    diagram of, 23
    location of, 4, 22

M

Mask, 74
Masseter muscle, 84
Mastoid process, 49
Medial pterygoid muscle, 84
Mentalis muscle, 81
Middle pharyngeal constrictor muscle, 61, 62
Mouth
    functions of, 59
    muscles of, 61–62, 80–81
Muscular process, 27
Mylohyoid muscle, 56, 57, 85

N

Nasal cavity, 75
Nasalis muscle, 76, 77
Nasopharynx, 60, 75
Nose, muscles of, 76–77
Nostrils, 75–77

O

Oblique arytenoid muscle, 36, 39
Omohyoid muscle, 50, 53, 58
Orbicularis oculi muscle, 78
Orbicularis oris muscle, 61, 81
Oropharynx, 60

P

Palate
    arching of, 66–67
    evolution and, 90–91
    function of, 63
    muscles of, 64–65
    sections of, 63
Palatoglossus muscle, 64, 65, 68, 69
Palatopharyngeus muscle, 49, 64, 65, 66
Passavant's cushion, 63
Pericardium, 10, 11
Pharyngeal tubercle, 61, 62
Pharynx
    evolution of, 94–95
    functions of, 59
    length of, 60
    muscles of, 61–62
    sections of, 60
    widened, 71
Piriform sinus, 28
Pleural cavity, 22
Posterior cricoarytenoid muscle, 36, 37, 42
Postural muscles, 17
Procerus muscle, 78, 79
Pterygomandibular raphe, 61
Pyramidalis nasi muscle, 78
Pyramid cartilages. *See* Arytenoid cartilages

Q

Quadratus lumborum muscle, 8

R

Rectus abdominis muscle, 14, 15, 18
Rhomboid major muscle, 20
Rhomboid minor muscle, 20
Ribs
    false, 3
    floating, 2, 3, 5
    joints of, 4–5
    movement of, 2, 6, 13, 17
    size of, 5
    true, 3
Risorius muscle, 81

S

Sacculus laryngis, 31
Sacrospinalis muscles, 17
Salpingopharyngeus muscle, 64, 65
Scalene muscles, 16
Scapulae, 20
Serratus posterior inferior muscle, 19
Serratus posterior superior muscle, 19
Singing
    arched palate and, 66
    expiratory muscles and, 13
    jaw's position during, 83
    suspensory muscles of the larynx during, 47,
        51–53, 71
    tongue's position during, 69–71
Spine
    support of, 17
    vertebrae of, 3
Sternocleidomastoid muscle, 16, 18
Sternohyoid muscle, 50, 52, 53, 54, 58
Sternothyroid muscle, 48, 49, 50, 52, 53, 58
"Strap" muscles, 58
Styloglossus muscle, 56, 57, 68, 69
Stylohyoid muscle, 50, 51, 54, 55
Styloid processes, 48, 49, 55
Stylopharyngeus muscle, 48, 49, 50, 52, 53, 71

Superior pharyngeal constrictor muscle, 61, 62
Superior thyroarytenoids, 30, 31
Swallowing, 47, 62, 63, 66, 88
Swimming, 63

T

Temporalis muscle, 84
Temporomandibular joint, 82–83
Tensor veli palatini muscle, 66
Thyroarytenoid muscle, 30, 31, 35, 41, 42, 92
Thyroepiglottic muscle, 31, 33
Thyrohyoid ligament, 48
Thyrohyoid membrane, 26
Thyrohyoid muscle, 48, 49, 50, 51, 53, 58
Thyroid cartilage, 26, 27, 28, 29, 31
Tidal flow, 24
Tongue
    anatomy of, 68–69
    false elevators of, 57
    functions of, 68–69
    position of, in singing, 69–71
Tongue bone. *See* Hyoid bone
Trachea, 22, 23, 31
Transverse arytenoid muscle, 36, 39
Transversus abdominis (transversalis) muscle, 15
Transversus thoracis muscle, 9, 14
Trapezius muscle, 21
Triticea cartilages, 26

U

Uvula, 64, 65, 66

V

Velum, 63
Ventricular bands, 30, 31, 92, 93
Vertebrae, 3
Vocal cords. *See* Vocal folds
Vocal folds
    in chest voice, 43
    design of, 92–93
    in falsetto, 46
    lengthening and shortening of, 37, 40–42
    location of, 31
    opening and closing of, 25, 26, 37–39
    structure of, 34
    wave action of, 42
Vocalis muscle, 30–31, 35, 41
Vocal ligaments, 26
Vocal processes, 27
Vocal production, five systems responsible for, xii, 97
Vocal tract, 59, 97

Z

Zygomaticus major muscle, 80, 81
Zygomaticus minor muscle, 80, 81

ABOUT THE AUTHOR

DR. THEODORE DIMON is the founder and director of The Dimon Institute and an adjunct professor at Teachers College, Columbia University. He received both master's and doctorate degrees in education from Harvard University and is an internationally renowned teacher of mind/body disciplines. He has written seven books, including *Anatomy of the Moving Body*; *The Body in Motion*; *Your Body, Your Voice*; *The Elements of Skill*; *The Undivided Self*; *A New Model of Man's Conscious Development*; and *Neurodynamics: The Art of Mindfulness in Action*.

ABOUT THE ILLUSTRATOR

G. DAVID BROWN has been the illustration program director at Winthrop University in South Carolina since 2005. Prior to that he was a medical illustrator for twenty-five years in Dallas, Texas. He completed his medical illustration graduate studies at the University of Texas Health Science Center at Dallas and his undergraduate studies in Visual and Environmental Studies at Harvard. This is the fifth book that he has illustrated with Ted Dimon.

ABOUT NORTH ATLANTIC BOOKS

NORTH ATLANTIC BOOKS (NAB) is an independent, nonprofit publisher committed to a bold exploration of the relationships between mind, body, spirit, and nature. Founded in 1974, NAB aims to nurture a holistic view of the arts, sciences, humanities, and healing. To make a donation or to learn more about our books, authors, events, and newsletter, please visit www.northatlanticbooks.com.